THE
Anti-Cancer,
Heart
Attack,
Stroke
DIET

THE
Anti-Cancer,
Heart
Attack,
Stroke
DIET

Bill Adler
and
Heather Harney

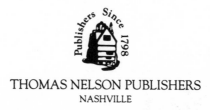

Publishers Since 1798

THOMAS NELSON PUBLISHERS
NASHVILLE

❖ *A Janet Thoma Book* ❖

Published in Nashville, Tennessee, by Thomas Nelson, Inc., and
distributed in Canada by Lawson Falle, Ltd., Cambridge, Ontario.

Library of Congress Cataloging-in-Publication Data
Adler, Bill.
    The anti-cancer, -heart attack, -stroke diet book / by Bill Adler and
Heather Harney.
       p.   cm.
    ISBN 0-8407-7119-3
       1. Cancer—Diet therapy—Recipes.   2. Coronary heart disease—Diet
therapy—Recipes.   3. Cerebrovascular disease—Diet therapy—
Recipes.   4. Salt-free diet.   5. Low-fat diet.   6. Low-cholesterol diet.
I. Harney, Heather.   II. Title.
RC271.D52A33   1991
641.5′63—dc20   90-49164
                                                                      CIP

Printed in the United States of America

1   2   3   4   5   6   7 — 96   95   94   93   92   91

Contents

Foreword by Richard E. Winter, M.D.

PART ONE
Diet Can Make a Difference Between Life and Death *1*

PART TWO
Three-in-One Recipes to Save Your Life *85*

APPENDICES *237*

NOTES

Foreword

Dr. Richard E. Winter
Chairman of Executive Health Group

DIET MAY MEAN the difference between life and premature death. Aside from cigarette smoking and driving while intoxicated, diet is the single most controllable element in postponing death. To modify a phrase, "You may become what you eat."

Many aspects of life over which we have no power affect us dramatically: airplane accidents and genetically controlled diseases, for example. If you knew that a certain plane flight was likely to crash, with a 25 percent chance of not arriving at its intended destination, would you take that flight? Certainly not. If you knew that eating a diet low in fried foods and high in fresh vegetables and whole grains, like cabbage, carrots, and oat bran, could decrease your chances of getting cancer by 25 percent, would you follow that kind of diet? Most likely, yes.

The only difference between plane flights and diet is knowledge. No one knows whether a particular flight is likely to crash, but you can be certain that a particular diet will significantly reduce the probability of your getting cancer. (Assigning an exact percent reduction is not possible.) Cancer and heart disease can be managed through diet.

But it wasn't always this way. The study of diet and health is a recent addition to the scope of modern medicine. The Framingham heart study, the first study to prove conclusively that fatty, salty diets multiply your risk of dying from stroke and heart attacks, originated in 1949. The first results were not available until the mid-1960s. Only in the past decade have physicians been aware of the relationship between particular foods and fatal diseases, such as fiber and colon cancer, oat bran and elevated cholesterol, fish and heart disease. Most of us were never taught by our parents or our schoolteachers about the relationship between diet and disease, because they were not aware of the connection. Our meals were prepared with taste, convenience and cost—not heart disease and cancer—in mind.

Science has advanced enough to be able to say what constitutes an anti-cancer, anti-heart disease diet. But that's not enough. Where science leaves off, and where *The Anti-Cancer, Heart Attack, Stroke Diet* begins, is in telling you about meals that are prepared not only with health in mind, but also with good taste, convenience and price in mind as well. In this book, science meets flavor.

As a physician and as chairman of Executive Health Group, I have the good fortune to be able to help thousands of men and women change their diet from a course that could condemn them to an early death from heart attack or cancer, to a diet that leads to longer, healthier and happier lives. Physicians may not be able to cure all forms of cancer, and we may not be able to repair a heart damaged by a heart attack. But if we can prevent these diseases, then we have accomplished our role as doctors.

Richard E. Winter, M.D.

Part One

Diet Can Make a Difference Between Life and Death

·1·

What in the World Can I Eat?

HAVE YOU EVER wandered through the supermarket, trying to pick foods that are "healthy"? The chore seems impossible. You feel as if you need a computer-like memory to recall all the foods and preservatives you shouldn't eat as well as the insight of a Ph.D. to combine all the diverse knowledge about the latest research. On one hand, you've heard that food additives are mostly harmful, but on the other, you remember that BHT, a preservative, might actually contribute to preventing cancer.

Or a recipe calls for asparagus, but the asparagus in the vegetable section looks as if it's suffering from advanced malnutrition: Will frozen asparagus be as good? What about substituting broccoli for asparagus? Which oil to buy? Never mind the fact that 90 percent of the food that grocery stores sell (in its marketed form, such as chicken with its skin) is unhealthy. Anything that comes in a package, processed or frozen, has a label listing ingredients. Vaguely you suspect that most of the ingredients with more than two syllables are bad for you and consequently try to avoid them, but you are still unsure if what you're buying promotes good health. Salt and sugar are listed as ingredients, too, but exact quantities remain a mystery. Formulating an anti-cancer, anti-heart attack, anti-stroke diet is like sailing a pleasure boat through the Strait of Hormuz.

And speaking of food: What about particular foods? Do peanuts promote cancer? Is all poultry safe? What's the best kind of beef to buy, if buying beef at all is a smart idea? What about celery, lima beans, and tofu? Is there much difference between skim and low-fat milk? Is *Jell-O* good or bad? Will a bag of *Doritos* take a year off your life?

And there's the Jekyll and Hyde food, the egg. Exactly how many eggs per week is healthy? What prepared foods like mayonnaise and breads contain egg yolks?

The questions are endless: Butter or margarine: is "buttering" bread ever a wise idea? Is eating fruit better than eating fiber cereal for breakfast? Does heating fruit and vegetables destroy their nutritional value? Nagging in the back of our minds are pieces of real information that we've heard on T.V. or read in the newspaper, such as fiber helping to reduce the occurrence of colon cancer. Alongside this information is another adage so ancient that it seems to be absolute truth: Eat a balanced diet from the four food groups: meat, vegetables, dairy, and carbohydrates.

Where is science when we really need it?

The more we know about nutrition—about preventing cancer and heart disease through diet—the more confusing is the preparation of a well-balanced meal.

The problem is not with the information, however; it is with how the information is presented. Science has given us ample research evidence to reduce the risk of heart attacks, strokes, arteriosclerosis, and cancer. That is, *using scientific insights, diet alone can dramatically reduce your chances of dying from cancer and heart disease.* If this is not apparent from reading articles about diet and health, it's because most articles report on only one specific aspect of health (for instance, the relationship between beta-carotene and cancer reduction). Most research linking diet to heart disease and cancer examines only a small aspect of the diet-health connection; if the article (or book) adopts a global approach, information concentrates on either cancer or heart disease prevention. Seldom are both treated adequately. Most of this research reports on particular studies; very little health reporting focuses on overall diet.

Regarding food, we as average Americans have an average amount of information about what we eat. We have enough information to cause us to wonder about, but not enough to answer, the question: "What can I eat?"

If you try to answer this question by buying cookbooks that offer low-cholesterol meals, you are left with the problem of figuring out how to prepare dinners that reduce your risk of cancer. If you buy a cookbook that touts anti-cancer meals, you find yourself wondering, "Are these recipes going to affect the health of my heart?" A visit to the bookstore usually leaves you with a thinner wallet, but not meals that will make you thinner and less prone to disease.

If you're more aggressive in figuring out what goes into an anti-cancer, anti-heart attack, anti-stroke menu, you could gather articles about healthful eating in newspapers and magazines. But these articles rarely provide concrete recipes and meal plans. In addition, they often report on narrowly defined research topics, providing incomplete or conflicting information.

On the other hand, you might discover an article telling you that fried food contributes to heart disease. Fine, that makes sense and is easy to comprehend. Just minimize fried foods in your diet. But another article might state that food fried in fish oil may help reduce the chance of heart attacks, and a third article might report that any fried food produces cancer-causing molecules. Yet another may say that broiling is better for your heart than frying, and still another will point out the fact that broiling makes certain food carcinogenic.

Perhaps microwaving is preferable food preparation. Or is boiling still the best way to cook? What happens to vitamins in the microwave or boiling pot?

The latest research may say that foods with beta-carotene are strongly anti-cancer, but how do you translate that research into practical meals? How do you reconcile data that shows vitamin A as being important in preventing cancer with medical warnings that too much vitamin A is harmful?

At this point you're ready to do one of two things: Become a strict vegetarian and remove yourself from the dinner circuit, or dine exclusively at McDonald's. Either is better than subjecting your brain to this storm of contradictory data.

That's where *The Anti-Cancer, Heart Attack, Stroke Diet* comes in. This book provides the synthesis of medical science's knowledge about nutrition, especially cancer and heart disease, and health. Most importantly, *The Anti-Cancer, Heart Attack, Stroke Diet* presents this information in a practical way: menus you can use.

If you've bought this book, you're already halfway along the road toward preventing cancer and heart disease. You've already decided that you are going to take an active, aggressive role in thwarting cancer and heart disease. (You are in the minority. The majority of Americans, alas, either don't recognize a connection between eating and preventing specific diseases, despite the frequency and thoroughness with which the media report on this, or they don't care.) You recognize that there is more than a statistical relationship between food and health: How you eat affects the progress of particular, deadly diseases. How you eat affects the quality and length of your life.

Diet is one aspect of a comprehensive approach toward preventing cancer and heart disease, and eight elements are a crucial part of such a plan:

- *Eat the right foods.* Concentrate on foods, for example, that have anti-cancer abilities or that lower blood cholesterol such as certain vegetables and oils.
- *Avoid foods that are dangerous.* These are almost too numerous to name, but include such junk food as hot dogs, cheeseburgers, candy, double-cheese pizzas, and bacon.
- *Avoid foods that are contaminated with pesticides and other toxins.* This involves carefully washing foods and trying to buy organic foods.
- *Supplement your diet with healthful activities* (exercise, keeping or developing a positive attitude toward life, and reducing stress).
- *Prepare foods wisely.* This is as important as what you eat.
- *Drink water,* a much overlooked "food," which can be significant in reducing your risk of disease.
- *Develop a program to lose weight* if you are obese. Obesity is strongly correlated with heart disease and cancer.
- *Stop smoking.* Right away. If you work or live around smokers, do whatever is in your power to change that.

Let's look at each of these components in turn.

EAT THE RIGHT FOODS

People fear cancer above all diseases, and rightfully so: No cancer is yet 100 percent curable for every individual, and many forms of cancer—lung cancer, bladder cancer, and stomach cancer—are among the most frightening diseases we know. But cancer is a strange disease, strange because, while medicine may not be able to cure many kinds of cancer, we have the knowledge and technology to help prevent many of these deadly cancers. As the chapter in the anti-cancer diet section shows, specific foods have strong anti-cancer properties. Carrots (specifically the beta-carotene in them) and cabbage contain chemicals that act to prevent cancer. As Jean Carper, author of *The Food Pharmacy* writes, "If we use chemotherapy to kill cancer cells after the fact, why not chemoprevention—the deliberate and controlled use of substances, including those abundant in foods, to block the effects of carcinogenic poisons around us—before the fact—before cancer has usurped the body."[1] Fiber is another cancer-preventing substance; although scientists are not entirely sure how fiber helps prevent colon cancer (possibly by speeding the passage of toxic material through the digestive system), they do know that it works.

Eating particular foods can act as an adjunct to a healthy heart. Onions raise the level of high density lipoproteins (HDLs) in the blood; HDLs are a good type of cholesterol that reduces the amount of bad cholesterol (low density lipoproteins, or LDLs) in your blood. Grains seem to have an effect on cholesterol, too: Rye, oats, and especially barley reduce the cholesterol level in the body. And not because they are fibrous, but because of the tocotrienol they contain which causes the liver to decrease the amount of cholesterol it produces. An oil called Omega-3, found in many fish, changes the body chemistry and seems to reduce the chance of heart attack. Olive oil, unlike other vegetable oils, lowers cholesterol levels, lowers blood pressure, and appears to retard cancer. Finally, eating the right kind of foods will ensure that you receive all the nutrients—amino acids, vitamins, carbohydrates and, yes, fats—your body needs.

AVOID DANGEROUS FOODS

Just as eating the right food is important, avoiding certain foods is equally crucial for good health. Keeping dangerous foods out of your system does not mean avoiding these foods all the time. Everyone likes to indulge once in a while, and the body seems to be able to cope with that. But it does mean eliminating certain foods and additives that are especially harmful. Excess salt, sugar, and fat top the list. Like rabbits left alone to multiply, these three "ingredients" form the basis for hundreds of foods, including, of course, the so-called (and aptly named) junk foods. The foods that contain too much salt, sugar, and fat are too numerous to list in one paragraph (or even an entire chapter!), but they are easy to spot. Pretty much everything served in fast food restaurants falls into this category; the same goes for all the foods you can buy by depositing two quarters in a vending machine. The salt shaker and sugar bowl are also a part of this regime. Salt and sugar content of other foods, however, is not necessarily as obvious. Coleslaw, a cabbage dish that can be an important part of your diet (some nutritionists maintain that one serving of coleslaw a week is enough to keep some cells from turning cancerous), has a dark side. Commercially prepared coleslaw often is filled with so much sugar that it could have been packaged by Hershey.

Other foods are more subtle. Chicken is a good source of protein and is a lean meat, but the skin is fatty. Beef, depending on the grade and cut, is marbled with fat. Stores that sell salads like to mix cheese and mayonnaise with the greens. Canned fruits are accompanied by sugary syrups. The bread you're buying may be made with plenty of salt or sugar. (The sugar may be in the form of honey, to make the bread sound healthier.) And buying breakfast cereals these days is like buying stock in a sugar mill.

Avoiding sugar, salt, and fat requires a little knowledge and a lot of vigilance. But the benefits are tremendous; one of those benefits is finding that foods are tastier than you had ever thought possible.

But salt, sugar, and fat aren't the only harmful additives that you should beware of. Modern agriculture and food processing wouldn't be possible without chemicals, including pesticides and preservatives. Not all additives are dangerous, however; just because a particular food contains a multi-syllabic ingredient doesn't mean that it is harmful. But sometimes it does. Some additives are universally dangerous, such as most pesticides. Other additives affect only certain individuals, such as monosodium glutamate (MSG) and sulfites. (The latter can cause death in sensitive individuals.) Some ingredients are probably inconsequential, but silly, like food coloring. Still others may actually enhance health, such as BHT, which some scientists speculate may retard cancer.

It's not the purpose of this book to examine food additives; that would be another entire book. But I'd like to stress two general rules of thumb regarding ingredients in your food. The fewer artificial-sounding ingredients in what you buy, the better. If you stick to that principle, you will be doing yourself a service. The number of additives a food has is also a good, general indicator of how processed that food is: the fewer the additives, the less the processing.

The second rule of thumb is to avoid pesticides. That's easy to say, but it seems hard to do because pesticides aren't listed as ingredients in the tomatoes, carrots, and limes you buy, even though the amount of pesticide residue on a particular vegetable may be greater than the amount of various additives that processed foods contain. In other words, store-bought fruits and vegetables can contain significant—dangerous—amounts of pesticide.

Before I tell you how to avoid pesticides, it's worthwhile knowing a little about why they are used so much and why they are so dangerous. Without doubt, pesticides have enabled farmers to increase their crop yields. Pesticides are also important when transporting produce across the country. Those little bugs love to munch while the vegetables are in warehouses or on trucks and trains. There's a great deal of controversy over whether pesticides are necessary, and over the amount of the pesticides we use. Regardless of your beliefs, however, there is no question that pesticides are toxic. They can cause cancer, birth defects, severe, irreversible damage to the immune system, allergic reactions, as well as induce sterility and reduce fertility. Many flu-like symptoms are not viral, but a consequence of pesticide exposure.

Almost every fruit and vegetable sprayed with pesticide retains some pesticide residue. In other words, always assume that cancer-causing chemicals linger on the "fresh" food you put in your shopping cart.

You should do everything possible to reduce the amount of pesticide in your food. First, look for organic produce that specifically says "pesticide free," which usually contains less pesticide than "commercial" produce. Because "organic" is a relative term, never hesitate to ask the produce manager where these vegetables were grown. By the way, vegetables with bruises and blemishes taste just as good as perfect-looking vegetables, and probably contain less pesticide. Often an inverse relationship exists between how a vegetable looks and how it tastes. Avoid out-of-season fruits and vegetables, which have more pesticide than in-season produce.

Local produce often contains less pesticide than fruits and vegetables shipped across the country, so try to buy locally grown foods. Farmers' markets are a good source for locally grown vegetables. Again, ask about the use of pesticides.

Foreign fruits contain the most pesticides. Other countries are not as stringent as the United States regarding use of pesticides. In fact, many pesticides that are illegal in the U.S. are exported to other countries, where they are used to prevent crop damage. Then those same fruits and vegetables containing the same illegal pesticides are shipped back to America.

Always wash vegetables thoroughly. Wash hard-skinned produce, such as pears, apples, and potatoes in a mildly soapy solution; then rinse off the soap. Peel the wax coating, which frequently contains fungicides, from fruits. Discard the outer leaves of lettuce and other leafy vegetables, which contain the most pesticides.

Unfortunately, it's impossible to avoid pesticides completely, which means you can't completely avoid cancer-causing (and other disease-causing) chemicals in your food. The best you can do is 1) reduce the amount of pesticide you consume, and 2) eat cancer-preventing foods.

WISE FOOD PREPARATION

How you prepare food is crucial. A raw carrot (peeled to remove residual pesticide) is the healthiest food you can eat. It's got fiber, beta-carotene, plenty of vitamins, it's low in calories, low in fat. But not so if the carrot is overcooked; then its vitamins and other nutrients disappear. And not so also if the carrot is cooked in a heavily salted broth, or a very creamy broth—the salt and fat may do more harm to your body than the carrot does good. Similarly, fish can be healthy. Its Omega-3 oils can reduce your chance of heart disease, but fish fried in butter or saturated oils falls into the unhealthy category. An occasional hamburger isn't bad, especially if it's lean beef, but a burger fried on a stove won't lose as much fat as a burger that's broiled. And a burger that's broiled on a barbecue, for example, may contain more cancer-causing chemicals than a burger that's cooked on a stove, because meats cooked over an open flame produce nitrosamines, a carcinogenic compound.

Sound confusing? It is—but only somewhat.

You can follow some guidelines to eliminate or reduce your risk of altering the beneficial effects of foods. First, for vegetables and fruits, the less cooking the better. Heat can destroy vitamins and other essential nutrients. (It goes without saying that frozen foods, even vegetarian foods, are, more often than not, completely robbed of many nutrients.) Cook at the lowest possible temperature and for the shortest amount of time. Surprisingly, microwave ovens, when used properly, do less damage to vegetables than boiling or steaming does.

Frying

Don't fry. Ever. Frying in butter or oil increases the fat content of foods. Even when you don't fry in butter, the fat has nowhere to go, and so it gets reabsorbed by the food. (This doesn't apply to stir-frying.) Fast-food potatoes come directly from a deep fryer and probably should only be consumed if you've been lost in the mountains for a week and they are the only food you can find. If you must fry, use a Teflon frying pan, and blot the food and pan with a paper towel as you cook, to remove the fat. Or, fry in a ridged pan, one that lets the fat drop onto a surface below the level of the meat.

In the same vein, don't cook with butter or saturated fats. Many recipes in traditional cookbooks include butter and oil because butter and oil are traditional. If you're worried about losing butter's flavor, keep in mind that cooking in butter doesn't necessarily add a buttery flavor to foods; the butter primarily keeps the food from sticking to the pan. Spices can give your recipes a flavor far tastier than butter ever gave them. If you're still worried about the food sticking to the pan, use Teflon, or a non-stick spray that contains little oil and few calories.

Broiling

Broiling may produce nitrosamines—cancer-causing compounds that forms when sodium nitrate or nitrite, two chemicals found in cured meats, react with amines. Broiling occasionally isn't too dangerous, but don't make broiled foods a staple of your diet.

DRINK WATER

The next component in your anti-cancer, anti-heart attack diet is water. Water is among the most important nutrients readily available. People can survive weeks without food, but without water we would expire in days. Every body process, from replenishing lost blood cells to digesting food, needs water. We lose water when we urinate and when we sweat. Marathon runners use up to five pounds of water weight during a race. Even during the coldest nights, sleeping causes us to lose water.

Besides keeping us away from the angel of death, water plays a part in preventing heart disease and cancer. First, the more water you drink, the less opportunity you have to eat a fatty french fry, or drink a chemical-laden soft drink. Water fills you up without any danger whatsoever. Today dozens of flavored waters, sparkling or non-carbonated, are on the market, so a glass of water is no longer an uninteresting, bland beverage. Depending on the brand you choose, water can be exciting, effervescent, and flavored with lime, orange, or even mixed berry. These flavors allow water to not only quench thirst, but to stave off appetite as well. Once you get into the habit, you're more likely to reach into your refrigerator for a glass of *Poland Spring* or *Perrier* than you are for some leftover chocolate cake. (How did that cake get into the fridge, anyway?)

Ah, the beauty of water. It's on your side when it comes to waging the battle of the bulge. A cup of ice cream (ah, so refreshing) has hundreds of calories contained mostly in fat; but a cup of water (equally refreshing) has no calories. So while you're drinking water, you are cutting back on calories. You're filling up, but not filling out.

Water has still more positive attributes. Drinking water helps keep your bowel movements regular, keeps your kidneys in working order, and helps maintain your body's proper metabolism.

DEVELOP A WEIGHT-LOSS PROGRAM

The recipes in *The Anti-Cancer, Heart Attack, Stroke Diet* are designed to help you reduce your risk of cancer and heart disease. One of the ways they work to accomplish the latter is by cutting back on calories. Calories are a target because, all other things being equal, the more calories you consume, the more obese you become. And the more you weigh, the greater your chance of a heart attack or stroke. When you are more than 30 percent heavier than your ideal weight, you have a greater chance of a shortened life span. Who says so? The American Heart Association and life insurance companies, who put their money where their statistics are. Fat people ("obese" is the preferred word, but "fat" is more accurate, more unpleasant to the ear, and more likely to impel someone to lose weight) have a greater ratio of LDLs to HDLs in their blood (the latter being associated with reduced risk of heart attack). The recipes in *The Anti-Cancer, Heart Attack, Stroke Diet* are designed to help you lose weight.

STOP SMOKING

Finally, smoking. It's hard to conceive of anything more likely to increase your risk of dying (or suffering unthinkable misery) from both heart disease and cancer. Maybe working in a coal mine without protective equipment, or removing asbestos from the ceiling of a fast-food restaurant that gives you free meals, but that's about it. Tobacco use kills, or more accurately, causes the premature death of, more Americans than any other single act. Each year cigarettes kill more Americans than car accidents, alcohol, cocaine, heroin, and AIDS combined. Over 300,000 Americans die from illness directly caused by smoking. Because of smoking, lung cancer has now surpassed breast cancer as the most common cancer in women. Middle-aged men and women who smoke suffer twice as many heart attacks as non-smokers. The list of smoking-induced diseases is large and could comprise an entire book. In short: If you smoke, quit. Because if you smoke, no amount of diet will have much effect on reducing your risk of cancer.

At the same time, it's important to avoid breathing other people's cigarette smoke. The Surgeon General has confirmed that passive smoking also causes cancer and heart disease. At least 5,000 cases of lung cancer each year are the result of secondary cigarette smoke. Request non-smoking sections when you eat in restaurants. If there aren't any designated areas, request a non-smoking section anyway; the restaurateur may get the idea. Also, ask your friends and family not to smoke around you. Smoking isn't as glamorous as it once was, and smokers usually put up with non-smoking requests.

The recipes in this book will bring you a long way toward a happier and healthier life. Remember, avoiding heart disease and cancer isn't just a matter of living longer; it's a matter of living happier. As your body becomes more resilient to cancer and heart disease through diet, you will feel better.

But what about eating out? The anti-cancer, anti-heart attack, and anti-stroke recipes in this book are marvelous, but you can't very well ask a restaurant owner if he'd mind your giving the chef a few lessons. Eating out is risky business, because often you don't know what goes on behind the kitchen's doors.

But you can follow certain precautions to eat more healthfully in restaurants. First, stay away from fast food chains: McDonald's, Burger King, Wendy's, Hardee's, and their companions in grease. The fat, salt, and sugar content in most fast foods is dangerously high. If you feel compelled to grab a quick bite at one of these places, eat one of their salads (go light on the salad dressing), or have an unadulterated burger—no bacon, no cheese, no special sauce.

Whenever you eat out, ask the waiter about the food on the menu. If you aren't sure whether something is fried, is cooked in butter, has mayonnaise in it, is made with saturated oils, or is sugar-laden, ask. The waiter may not know, but he can ask the cook, who will probably be delighted that somebody is interested in what goes into his menu. If they don't know, you probably shouldn't be eating what they're serving anyway. The real key to maintaining your anti-cancer, anti-heart attack, anti-stroke diet is being alert to what you're eating.

Many restaurants now have "lite" and low-cholesterol meals on their menus. If you find a restaurant with these selections, your work is done for you. Most of the time you can order freely from them.

Avoid fried foods. Even fish, normally a healthy food, becomes unhealthy when fried. Request your fish broiled, poached, or baked instead of fried. Treat other fried foods in the same way.

Avoid sauces on your meals. If the menu says "with chef's sauce," ask politely to hold the sauce. Same for mayonnaise.

Eat salads. A hearty salad before the meal will reduce your appetite. But a good salad can be turned into a fattening, artery-hardening course by its dressing. Creamy, buttery, and cheesy dressings essentially make your salad unhealthy. Avoid them. Instead use light vinaigrettes or oil and vinegar (with an emphasis on the vinegar).

Other good-for-you appetizers include fresh fruit, shrimp (not cooked in butter), and other non-smoked fish. It takes about twenty minutes for food that you eat to register in your brain's hunger center, so allow that much time between your appetizer and the beginning of the meal.

Eliminate the butter from your table. If you have enough will power, don't butter your bread; if your grit isn't that strong, ask the waiter to remove the butter. Consider telling the waiter not to even bring bread to your table.

The same goes for ketchup. Considerable quantities of salt and sugar have been added to ketchup. A preferable and tasty alternative is to place a slice of tomato on your food, rather than pouring a layer of ketchup. As a condiment, ketchup has a role to play on sandwiches, burgers, and other foods, but when used as a coating for food, ketchup adds hundreds of calories and milligrams of salt to your diet.

Last, beware the salt shaker. Most restaurant foods are already spiced professionally by the chef, so salting your food is unnecessary. Yet most people salt their food out of habit. If your habit is strong, ask the waiter to remove the salt shaker from your table. (Is there anything left? Of course, that healthful glass of water!)

Above all, use common sense. Pay attention to what you're eating. Most dinners can be modified to your liking. After all, restaurants are supposed to serve *you,* the customer.

The guidelines suggested in this overview are borne out by evidence cited in the Surgeon General's report, which is summarized in the next chapter. In the next three chapters we will look at these three diseases individually, giving you general guidelines for reducing your susceptibility to each of them. Then, in Chapter 5, we will show you how exercise can help prevent these three diseases. Finally, in Chapter 6, chef Heather Harney will give you some general guidelines for "three-in-one" cooking, which will reduce your susceptibility to all three diseases at the same time. Part Two of the book will present 160 recipes that were especially created by Heather to provide this "three-in-one" protection.

·2·

Anti-Cancer Diet

BY THE YEAR 2000, two out of five people in America will develop some form of cancer.

This year alone, almost one million new cancer cases will be diagnosed.

Even as you read this book, a woman will die of breast cancer *every fifteen minutes.*[1]

No wonder then that in a recent *Washington Post*–ABC News survey, cancer topped the list of diseases Americans hope never to get—surpassing AIDS and heart disease as the country's most dreaded illness.[2]

So far, scientists have battled courageously and unceasingly to isolate the *cause* of cancer and have failed. Nor have they been able to pinpoint any specific *cure* for the disease. The good news is that through the years a certain degree of control has been developed over the disease. Treatment usually involves radical surgery and/or painful radiation therapy with sometimes unpredictable and toxic side effects.

But things are changing for the better.

LOOKING ON THE BRIGHT SIDE

Quite recently scientists have estimated that approximately one-third of all cancers are diet-related and may be prevented by controlling the foodstuffs you eat. Three important voices have proclaimed this vital role for nutrition in the prevention of cancer:

- Dr. Richard Rivlin, chief of Nutrition Services at Memorial Sloan-Kettering Cancer Center in New York City
- Dr. Peter Greenwald of the National Cancer Institute
- Dr. Charles LeMaistre of the American Cancer Society

Dr. Rivlin warns that cancer is not a single disease with a single cause, but depends on genetics, lifestyle (including alcohol intake, physical activity, and smoking), and diet as well. Drs. Greenwald and LeMaistre agree that diet is an important environmental factor that may reduce certain risks of cancer, particularly cancer of the gastrointestinal tract.[3]

CORRELATIONS BETWEEN DIET AND CANCER

Although no cause-effect relationship has yet been proven, correlations have been found between diet and cancer. If indeed the implementation of certain diets and combinations of foods can reduce the average person's risk of contracting cancer, then we can say that we have moved one giant step closer to the eradication of this most feared of all modern civilization's diseases.

Certainly, prevention of any disease is preferable to cure. For that reason alone, Americans give highest priority to nutritional research in the area of cancer prevention.

New information is being amassed and compiled daily. Research is going on in a wide nutritional area. As yet, no new and startling treatment has been found that will totally eliminate this dreadful disease. But a foundation for the better management of cancer has been developed and is being perfected.

SEVEN GUIDELINES TO AN ANTI-CANCER DIET

Accordingly, the National Cancer Institute recently released seven interim dietary guidelines that may help reduce your chances of cancer. They involve these basic elements of diet:

1. Avoid obesity.
2. Reduce the amount of total fat intake.
3. Eat more high-fiber foods.
4. Eat more foods rich in vitamin A and vitamin C.
5. Eat more cruciferous vegetables.
6. Moderate your intake of salt-cured, smoked, and nitrite-cured foods.
7. Moderate your consumption of alcohol.[4]

Let's take up these seven guidelines one by one.

1. Avoid Obesity

According to National Cancer Institute findings, you should provide for yourself a varied, well-balanced diet, with the addition of regular exercise, to help you achieve and maintain an ideal weight. The N.C.I. further advises that you eat in moderation to keep your weight down, since obesity is associated with cancer of the breast, colon, uterus, gallbladder, and stomach.

Cheryl Loggins, president of the California Dietetic Association, long an advocate of dieting to prevent cancer, echoes the N.C.I. call for moderation:

"Another step up the health ladder is to keep the word 'moderation' in mind," she says. "Moderate portion sizes and moderate intake of extra foods: in the short run it will help keep your weight at a reasonable level; in the long run, you'll be healthier and more active and you'll feel better."[5]

2. Reduce the Amount of Total Fat Intake

The intake of fat and cancer were linked in early studies on rats, studies from as early as the 1920s when Albert Tannenbaum of the Michael Reese Hospital in Chicago discovered and established a definite association of dietary fat with breast cancer.

Later in the 1960s, analysis of diseases in various countries and epidemiological studies by Kenneth K. Carroll of the University of Western Ontario and Ernest L. Wynder of the American Health Foundation established a definite link between the intake of dietary fat and death from breast cancer.

Experiments on laboratory animals conducted by N.C.I.'s Greenwald and Drs. Wynder and John Weisburger of the American Health Foundation have recently confirmed the findings of those earlier studies. It is now an established fact that the lower the fat intake of the rat, the fewer and smaller the breast tumors that result.[6]

A Pervasive Medical Bias

Why weren't these findings immediately put into circulation to involve all women?

Victoria Leonard, executive director of the National Women's Health Network, claims that a bias exists in the medical profession against regulating nutrition to prevent breast cancer.

"They think women won't follow a low-fat diet," she states. She also says that women need counseling to change their high-fat intake. "We are saying, give us the information and let us make the choice. Tell us what the risks are and let us decide."[7]

One study initiated to discover correlations between fat intake and breast cancer was that performed by the Harvard Medical School on ninety thousand nurses. That study revealed no such linkage. However, Ms. Leonard pointed out that this particular study was based on a figure of 30 percent fat intake; other studies based on a 20 percent fat intake, she said, showed a definite *decrease* in the growth of breast cancer. "The average American diet is 40 percent fat," Ms. Leonard observes.[8]

A pamphlet issued by the National Women's Health Network suggests that cancer-conscious women reduce the fat in meat, dairy products, and vegetable oils, except perhaps olive oil and Omega-3 oils found in some fish.

New Experiments Now Ongoing

The National Cancer Institute is now conducting a long-term low-fat study to determine whether diets containing 20 percent or less of total calories from fat will reduce the incidence of breast cancer in women.

N.C.I.'s Greenwald has a tip on cutting down on fat intake. "Take your usual diet—the one that you are happy with—and go through the different food groups and cut down on the fat in each one of them. If you do that, you will get down to 30 percent fat."[9]

John Dickerson, professor of human nutrition at Surrey University in England, has noted that excessive intake of fat could raise the levels of prolactin and other breast hormones and might thus be responsible for changes in the structure of mammary tissue that could lead to cancer of the breast:

I believe it may be possible by dietary manipulation, particularly by reducing fat in the diet, to manipulate prolactin and estrogens to prevent breast cancer, particularly among women otherwise at high risk of the disease.[10]

In general, N.C.I. study guidelines indicate that Americans should reduce their fat intake, both saturated and polyunsaturated, from the current average of about 40 percent of total calories daily to about 30 percent or less. In addition, the guidelines say that cutting down on fat and caloric intake helps control body weight. High-fat diets, the guidelines add, seem to be a factor in cancers of the breast, colon, and prostate.

3. Eat More High-Fiber Foods

"Fiber" consists of a group of substances in plants that is partly or not digestible. A number of foods are high in this type of fiber, including whole-grain breads and cereals, fruits and vegetables, and beans (known as "legumes" in nutrition circles).

N.C.I.'s Greenwald comments on fibers:

> I think that if you take the diet in moderation, just increase the fiber and cut down on the fat and keep trim, that's about all that we can really say. We think that making these changes will reduce the risk of cancer of the colon, cancer of the breast, perhaps cancer of the prostate, and perhaps several other things.[11]

David Kritchevsky, associate director of the Wistar Institute in Philadelphia and a leading researcher on dietary fiber, issues a slight disclaimer on fibers:

> We definitely need more fiber in our diets, but it is not a magic medicine that is going to keep cancer away. Listen carefully to all those television commercials. The qualifying word is "may."[12]

Nevertheless, fiber intake does help fight cancer, he says:

> All the associations between cancer and fiber have been from epidemiological studies. These studies have shown populations with a high fiber diet have lower incidences of colon cancer.[13]

Richard S. Rivlin, chief of Nutrition Services at Memorial Sloan-Kettering Cancer Center, has even speculated on the reason fiber acts to keep cancerous substances out of the bodily system:

> Since fiber is not broken down by enzymes, it passes through the body easily and sort of acts like a clean sweep. It accelerates the rate in which substances, including carcinogens, pass through the tract. Remember, this is conjecture on our part. No one knows for sure exactly how fiber is beneficial.[14]

How Much Fiber in a Diet?

A good high-fiber diet would be somewhere between twenty-five and thirty-five grams a day. Such a diet, it should be noted, is usually low in fat and calories, which could in turn promote weight loss.

4. Eat More Foods Rich in Vitamin A and Vitamin C

Plant foods that are rich in vitamin A (actually beta-carotene, which *becomes* vitamin A once it is in the body) may help prevent cancer. Such plant foods include dark green leafy vegetables and deep yellow fruits and vegetables like carrots, spinach, broccoli, peppers, winter squash, sweet potatoes, peaches, apricots, and cantaloupes.

Fruits like oranges, grapefruits, strawberries, melons, papayas, mangos, and kiwi fruits also contain vitamin C. Vegetables rich in vitamin C include broccoli, cauliflower, and peppers. Vitamins A and C may lower the risk of cancer of the larynx, esophagus, stomach, and lungs.

A recent study at Johns Hopkins School of Hygiene and Public Health in Baltimore showed that a diet of vegetables and grains high in beta-carotene appeared to decrease the risk of lung cancer. On the other hand, people with low levels of beta-carotene in their blood were about four times more likely to develop squamous cell carcinoma, a common form of lung cancer.

Something Protective in Beta-Carotene

"There appears to be something in the diet that is protective," points out Marilyn Menkes, an epidemiologist at Johns Hopkins, in discussing beta-carotene. "I don't think it would hurt people, and it might help them, to improve their diet [in vitamin A]. That is, eat more leafy, dark green vegetables, whole grains, and bran."[15]

A study by the American Cancer Society's Lawrence Garfinkel supported the society's recommendations of fruits and vegetables and other foods rich in beta-carotene. He says:

I think this study is a very valuable addition to the literature. Our feeling is that if you eat a good balanced diet, you get all the beta-carotene you need.[16]

Cancers of the Colon

Colorectal cancer is the third most common form of cancer in the United States, with 130,000 new cases diagnosed every year. Sixty thousand colon cancer deaths occur annually; it is the second leading form of cancer death in men and the third leading cause among women, especially in adults over the age of fifty.

Dr. Emily White, a scientist in the Cancer Prevention Research Unit at the Fred Hutchinson Cancer Research Center says: "People with a high vegetable diet have a significantly lower risk of colorectal cancer."[17]

5. Eat More Cruciferous Vegetables

Cruciferous vegetables are those of the *Cruciferae* family, the family that includes, most commonly, cabbage and mustard. Some substance found in vegetables of this kind—cabbage, broccoli, cauliflower, bok choy, brussels sprouts, kale, collard greens, rutabagas, turnips, and kohlrabi—protects against cancer of the gastrointestinal tract and respiratory tract. Little is known conclusively regarding how cruciferous vegetables reduce cancer risk.

6. Moderate Your Intake of Salt-cured, Smoked, and Nitrite-cured Foods

Your risk of cancer of the esophagus and stomach may be increased by eating too much smoked fish, poultry, meat, and nitrite-containing foods like bacon, sausage, frankfurters, ham, and luncheon meats.

There is a very good reason for this fact. Chemicals produced in the smoking process may become cancerous when the food so processed finally metabolizes in the bodily system. Nitrites that prevent botulism and act as color preservatives for foodstuffs can combine with protein in the body to form dangerous nitrosamines.

The N.C.I. recommends eating fresh, unprocessed fish, poultry, and lean meats, and moderating as much as possible the intake of salt-cured, smoked, and nitrite-cured foods.

7. Moderate Your Consumption of Alcohol

One or two drinks daily of beer, wine, or cocktails is considered a moderate amount of alcoholic consumption. However, excess alcohol intake, particularly for smokers, can be linked with cancer of the liver, mouth, throat, larynx, and esophagus.

Dr. Tim Byers of the State University of New York at Buffalo has found another connection. Alcoholic consumption may be related to breast cancer, he says. Citing fourteen studies, he points out that all report some correlation between alcohol consumption and breast cancer in women. Most of the studies show that the incidence of cancer increases with the frequency and amount of alcohol consumed.[18]

Another study in Boston reports that the women in the sample who drank at least four times a week were two-and-a-half times as likely to get breast cancer as nondrinkers.

GENERAL RULES OF DIET TO PREVENT CANCER

"Using a proper diet as an effective weapon against your risk for disease involves just that: the total diet," CDA's Loggins says. "The California Dietary Association recommends eating for good health in general. That translates into eating a daily variety of foods from the nutrient-based food groups."[19]

Such a diet should include foods from each of the four main groups for every meal, accompanied by appropriate liquids. Here are some of them, selected from these groups, with the daily servings recommended by the American Cancer Society's diet guidelines:

- *Milk and Milk Products.* Foods from the dairy group include cheese and yogurt. DAILY RECOMMENDATION: 2 to 4 servings. SERVING SIZE: 1 cup low-fat milk, cottage cheese, or yogurt; 1½ ounces cheddar cheese.
- *Meat, Fish, Poultry, and Alternates.* Alternates in this meat group include peanut butter, low-fat cheese, beans, and lentils. DAILY RECOMMENDATION: 2 servings. SERVING SIZE: 2 to 3 ounces cooked lean meat, poultry, or fish; 4 tablespoons peanut butter; 1 cup cooked dried peas, beans, or lentils; 2 ounces cheddar or cottage cheese; 2 eggs (but not to exceed 3 eggs a week!). NOTE: Three ounces of cooked meat means a piece of sirloin steak about 4 × 2 × ½ inches.
- *Breads and Cereals.* Foods from this cereal group include rice, muffins, and pasta. DAILY RECOMMENDATION: 3 to 5 servings. SERVING SIZE: 1 slice of bread, muffin, or roll; ½ to 1 cup cereal, cooked rice, or macaroni.
- *Fruits and Vegetables.* Foods from this group include green and

deep yellow vegetables. DAILY RECOMMENDATION: 4 or 5 servings. SERVING SIZE: 1/2 cup.
• *Liquids.* This includes beverages, juices, and soups. DAILY RECOMMENDATION: 8 to 12 cups of liquid, in general. SERVING SIZE: Any amount desired.

At the same time you are paying attention to the foodstuffs mentioned above, you should also be noting your intake of fats, and reducing your consumption of gravies, sauces, sweets, sodas, and chips.

The Value of Moderation in Food Intake

Michael Pariza of the University of Wisconsin at Madison points out that cutting back on total caloric intake—that is, adopting moderation in everything, including everything you eat and drink—would mean "better-balanced diets because people will be able to pursue a wider range of nutritional options in their efforts to prevent cancer. For instance, it may not be necessary to trim away every last morsel of fat from your meat so long as you reduce your calorie count in some other way—say, eating less sweets."

In fact, he says, "Our rat experiments indicate that a small restriction in calories can have a major impact in reducing cancer. That could potentially have enormous bearing on the human population."[20]

Decreasing Fat in Recipes

The person preparing foods for the family can reduce the amount of fat used in cooking in a number of ways.

In recipes, for example, you can reduce the amount of eggs, butter, margarine, oil, and mayonnaise used. Simply pare the original amounts to one-half or three-quarters. Instead of using creamy salad dressing, use a reduced-calorie dressing such as vinegar or lemon juice. As much as possible, substitute low-fat or nonfat (skim) milk, low-fat cheese, plain low-fat yogurt, and buttermilk for whole milk, cheese, sour cream, and heavy cream.

Soft cheeses are usually lower in fat content than hard cheeses. Cottage cheese, pot cheese, farmer cheese, part-skim ricotta, and part-skim mozzarella are usually more desirable than cheddar, American, Swiss, and parmesan. The one exception is cream cheese, which is soft, but unexpectedly high in fat.

Replace heavy cream or whipped cream in recipes with evaporated skim milk. To reduce the amount of mayonnaise in sandwiches, substitute mustard or reduced-calorie mayonnaise.

Cutting Fat Out of Your Foods

Begin to serve skinless poultry, veal, fish, and lean cuts of meat. Before you cook, trim all visible fat. Then, when serving, limit your portions of meat to small pieces: three to four ounces of cooked meat per person. When serving tuna fish, use water-packed tuna, not oil-packed.

Put more fiber in your diet by serving a variety of high-fiber foods like fruits and vegetables, especially those rich in vitamins A and C. Use beans, lentils, seeds, and peas in casseroles, soups, stews, dips, and salads. Instead of serving refined breads, choose whole wheat, bran, pumpernickel, oatmeal, or corn breads, crackers, and muffins.

Instead of sweetened low-fiber cereals, use bran cereals, oatmeals, or shredded wheat. When baking, use whole wheat flour for some or all of the white flour. In addition, make pancakes, tortillas, or pasta out of whole wheat flour, not white flour.

In topping casseroles, use a mixture of bread crumbs and bran or wheat germ. Other good sources of fiber are brown rice and other cooked grains like barley, millet, bulgur, and buckwheat (sometimes called "kasha").

Cooking to Beat Cancer

Don't fry foods; instead, bake, roast (with rack), boil, steam, oven-broil, stew, poach, stir-fry, or microwave them. These methods require the use of little or no additional fat. When you sauté or stir-fry, use a nonstick skillet that requires no fat. When you roast meat, cook at a low temperature and place a rack in the pan to let the fat drip below the meat so that fat can be drained before serving. When you cook with a steamer, use the double-boiler type, or one with a basket. Use a heavy Dutch oven if possible for steady, even cooking.

Flavor with herbs, spices, onions, garlic, vinegar, ginger, lemon juice, mustard, wine, broth, fruit juice, or vegetable sauce rather than with high-fat cream sauce and gravy. If you do require a gravy, refrigerate it before you serve it, and discard the solid fat that rises to the top just before eating it.

Cook vegetables quickly, and remove them from the heat when they are tender-crisp. Use as little water as possible in cooking, and bring to a boil before adding vegetables. Use leftover cooking liquids in stews and soups. Cook with as few liquids as you can.

Use a vegetable purée as a sauce rather than a butter-based sauce. Instead of thickening a sauce with flour, use cornstarch; then you won't have to use any extra fat as you do with flour.

Tips on Barbecuing, Grilling, and Broiling

When you barbecue, grill, or broil meat, you may be endangering yourself with a possibly cancerous chemical—benzopyrene —that forms from the smoke and flames. You can limit this potential danger by doing the following:

1. Cook lean meats slowly at a low temperature.
2. Do not overcook any meat.
3. Move racks or grills as far away as possible from the source of the heat.
4. Wrap food in foil, or put it in a pan before grilling or barbecuing.

Choosing the "Right" Food over the "Wrong"

One of the best ways to adhere to the American Cancer Society's Diet Guidelines is to teach yourself to choose the "right" food over the "wrong." A look at the calories in the chart below should give you a good idea of *why* you should make the proper choice. For example, instead of choosing a doughnut (235 calories), choose a plain muffin (120 calories).

More of these interesting choices follow:

AVOID	CAL	CHOOSE	CAL
fried chicken (3 oz. dark meat with skin)	240	roast chicken (3 oz. white meat without skin)	145
rib roast (4 oz.)	300	lean flank steak (4 oz.)	200
spare ribs (4 oz.)	450	lean pork tenderloin (4 oz.)	275
whole milk (1 cup)	150	skim milk (1 cup)	85
mayonnaise (2 tbs.)	120	low-cal mayonnaise (2 tbs.)	40

chocolate cake, iced		angel food cake, plain	
(1 piece)	310	(1 piece)	121
ice cream (1/2 cup)	135	low-fat yogurt (1/2 cup)	75
peanuts (1/2 cup)	420	plain popcorn (2 cups)	108

Eating Out the "Right" Way

Dining out on the town or eating out when you travel can have a disastrous effect on your best dietary intentions. But not necessarily. With a bit of insight and planning, you can easily conform to your intended guidelines. Here are some suggestions on how to do so:

- If you overindulge for one special occasion, eat moderately for several days after.
- Eat at restaurants featuring low-calorie or light meals.
- Ask to have a fried dish steamed or broiled.
- Beware of high-fat foods; concentrate instead on fruits, vegetables, and whole-grain foods.
- Order salad or soup rather than an entrée.
- Choose clear soups over cream soups.
- Order salads with dressing on the side so you can serve yourself.
- Split a dish, or several dishes, with your dining companion.
- Choose fish or chicken dishes over beef and pork dishes.
- Cut all visible fat off meats before eating.
- Use butter sparingly on rolls or bread.
- Don't eat sautéed or deep-fried foods.

Menu Suggestions for Anti-Cancer Dieting

The following combinations can be used for typical anti-cancer meals:

BREAKFAST

Whole-grain, unsweetened cereal, sliced fruit, and low-fat milk. Fruit with low-fat cottage cheese. Buckwheat pancakes topped with fruit. Poached egg with Canadian bacon (lower in fat than regular bacon) and whole wheat toast. Bran or English muffin with fruit preserves.

LUNCH

Minestrone, lentil, or split pea soup. Green salad (omit bacon bits, cheese, and cold cuts) with vinaigrette dressing. Fruit with low-fat yogurt. Turkey, chicken, or tuna fish sandwich without mayonnaise. Baked potato topped with spinach or low-fat plain yogurt and chives. Vegetarian chili.

DINNER

Fresh or marinated vegetables, fruit cup, or seafood cocktail. Fish, poultry (no skin), or lean meat that is baked, roasted, poached, or steamed. Pasta, served with a vegetable sauce like tomato. Steamed vegetables without butter or cheese sauce. Starches like a baked or boiled potato, brown rice, or whole wheat pasta. Whole-grain enriched breads, bread sticks, crackers, or muffins.

DESSERTS

Fresh fruit, fruit compote, sherbet, sorbet, fruit ices, fruited gelatin, ice milk, frozen low-fat yogurt, or angel food cake. Beverage options: skim or low-fat milk, citrus fruit juices, vegetable juices, and sparkling waters.

FAST FOODS

Plain lean hamburger or lean roast beef. Roast chicken or baked fish without breading. Pizza topped with part-skim mozzarella cheese and vegetables like green peppers. Baked potato topped with cottage cheese (preferably low-fat). Corn on the cob without butter. Bean tacos or bean chili.

IN GENERAL

Try to include more fruits, vegetables, whole grains, legumes, low-fat dairy products, poultry, fish, and lean meat in your menus.

Outwit Cancer? Do Something About It!

Central to the whole idea of eating to outwit cancer is this: "It's one thing for people to be aware of the information available on diet. It's another thing for people to *do* something about it."[21] So says Irving Irmer, spokesperson for the American Cancer Society. He adds that it will take a "substantial educational effort to bring about change" in diet to effect cancer prevention.[22]

Irmer speaks from experience. The American Cancer Society has found that, even though 80 percent of Americans believe that a diet high in fresh fruits, vegetables, and fiber may help prevent cancer and that a diet high in red meat and cured or smoked fish or meats may help promote cancer, only 15 percent of the population has changed its eating habits accordingly.[23]

A Ready Reference

The anti-cancer menus are designed to serve as quick references for adequate food intake. (Note that all recipes are designed to serve one person.) They include well-balanced meals that may not only allow you to reduce your family's risk of getting cancer, but will also help you to maintain a state of everyday fitness.

There are one hundred recipes in the anti-cancer section of the book, containing a variety of different foodstuffs to be prepared and eaten throughout the year. These preferences form an interesting and attractive diet, suitable for all families.

·3·

Anti-Heart Attack Diet

ALMOST ONE-HALF of the deaths in the United States are caused by some form of cardiovascular disease, usually a stroke or a heart attack. Certain risk factors exist that increase the likelihood of a stroke or a heart attack, factors that are involved in diet, heredity, age, and habits of living.

For example, anyone addicted to cigarette smoking is likely to sustain a stroke or heart attack. People who do not exercise enough and who are overweight are more likely to be victims of heart attacks or strokes than those who exercise and control their weight.

On the other hand, women until menopause seem to be protected from heart attack, as compared to men in the same age grouping. Heredity is also a definite risk factor: if your parents have died of heart attacks, you are likely to follow suit. The likelihood of your suffering a heart attack or stroke also increases with your age.

IMPORTANT RISK FACTORS IN HEART DISEASE

The three highest risk factors in early heart attack have been identified in extensive studies of cardiovascular disease performed in Framingham, Massachusetts, the "Framingham Studies," in which more than 5,000 men and women aged thirty to sixty years were involved.

These three high-risk factors are:

1. An elevation of cholesterol in the blood.
2. An elevation in blood pressure (hypertension).
3. Cigarette smoking.

Lesser risks are:

4. An elevation of triglycerides in the blood.
5. Diabetes mellitus.
6. Lack of exercise.
7. Obesity.
8. Excessive stress.

Of all these eight factors, the most important to the average person is the elevation of cholesterol in the blood. This section of the book will deal with cholesterol and how to control your cholesterol level by what you eat and drink.

WHAT CHOLESTEROL REALLY IS

The typical dictionary defines cholesterol: "A steroid alcohol $C_{27}H_{45}OH$ present in animal cells and body fluids, important in physiological processes, and implicated experimentally as a factor in arteriosclerosis."

The dictionary definition addresses the fundamental condition of arteriosclerosis: its probable involvement in the hardening of the arteries ("arterio" = of the arteries; "sclerosis" = hardening).

Cholesterol is critical in a medical sense because a high level in the bloodstream increases the risk of heart disease by coating and clogging the inner surface of the arteries. The good news is that, if you know your blood cholesterol level and realize that it is too high, you can reduce the risk of heart disease by lowering it. And you can do it with simple dietary measures!

The following profile of a cholesterol describes its nature and function in the body:

Cholesterol is a "lipid"—a fat-like substance also called a blood fat—that is employed by the human body to manufacture essential components of the bodily system such as cell walls, bile acids, protective sheaths around nerve fibers, vitamin D, and body hormones.

Cholesterol is carried in the blood, along with protein, in packages that are called "lipoproteins"—fat-like proteins.

Enough cholesterol to repair cell membranes and nerve sheaths and to make acids, vitamin D, and hormones can be regularly produced in the liver. Obviously, little motivation remains for ingesting cholesterol to assist in body maintenance.

An Important Building Block

Thus cholesterol is one of nature's building blocks, used for several specific and essential purposes in the body. However, it is also present in the bodies of other forms of life, including animals and animal products that are eaten by human beings for nourishment. When the outside cholesterol enters the human bloodstream, it tends to become an added substance that may not be needed by the body at all.

For example, it is now known that the human body manufactures about 600 milligrams of cholesterol every day, to take care of cell wall and nerve sheath repair and the production of hormones, vitamin D, and bile acids. The amount of cholesterol manufactured naturally is more than adequate for the typical human being's needs.

And yet the average American consumes about 1,000 milligrams of cholesterol every day, 400 milligrams more than the body manufactures! Thus, at any one given time, the body has a superabundance of cholesterol.

The Problem with Building Blocks

Cholesterol's role in repairing cell membranes and in manufacturing hormones, bile acids, and vitamin D is a virtual necessity for the maintenance of good health. When cholesterol is present in great abundance, however—that is, when you've got too much of it in your system—it can be the cause of trouble that in the end can be fatal.

Remember that this building material is insoluble in blood. It is waxy and slippery, and when it is too much in evidence it tends to accumulate wherever it can.

Not being needed, it has no place to go but out. And getting out is not quite so easy as it might seem. There are lengthy corridors in the arterial system that must be traversed before an exit can be found. The cholesterol blocks simply slow down, are pushed aside by the blood, and settle onto the inner surface of the arteries. There they cling and harden, causing "hardening" of the arteries. They become "atherosclerotic deposits"—("athero" = by chaff or waste; "sclerotic" = hardening).

How Arterial Blood Clotting Starts

When cholesterol settles on the arterial surfaces, the smooth-muscle cells of the artery walls are stimulated to multiply. The buildup of cholesterol may even damage the muscle cells themselves or other structures in the arterial walls.

Once these cells are injured, they become dislodged from the artery wall, leaving raw tissue exposed to the bloodstream. This tissue, called "collagen," attracts platelets (certain blood cells) which accumulate on the surface of the arterial walls. This gathering of platelets forms a mass of material known as a "blood clot."

The clotting of blood from these platelets may eventually form an accumulation massive enough to block the artery and stop the normal flow of blood. Such blood clots, depending on where in the arterial system they form, can cause heart attacks or strokes.

Accumulation of Dangerous Debris

When the smooth-muscle cells, under the stimulation of cholesterol deposits, multiply and move into the artery wall, they form a fibrous network called "plaque." This network becomes a lesion that contributes to the process of atherosclerosis, the hardening of the artery walls from accumulated "chaff" or debris, including injured cells. In addition, cholesterol's building blocks help intensify this dangerous layer of plaque. All this material—cells, connective tissue, cholesterol, and the debris from dying cells—piles up steadily on the surface of the artery wall. Soon the thickness may protrude into the passageway of the artery proper, in some instances totally obstructing the flow of vital blood through the artery.

Plaque can sometimes appear in the coronary arteries, eventually causing chest pains (angina pectoris), which occur when too little blood and oxygen is allowed to reach the heart muscle. This sensitive muscle may die from the lack of nourishment by oxygen. A heart attack (myocardial infarction) may result.

Atherosclerosis, the steady degeneration of the arterial cells and accumulation of dead cells and cholesterol blocks, can progress at a slow but steady pace, quite unnoticed. It can also develop rapidly. The damage it causes may vary from a simple arterial coating to a blocked artery.

No Place to Go

In this way, plaque and other deposits in the walls of the coronary vessels of the heart may eventually lead to heart attacks and strokes. Once the surface of the inner artery becomes damaged by plaque, the available area for blood flow becomes constricted. With the narrowed diameter of the artery preventing a full flow of blood, the heart must strain and pump harder to push life-giving blood through the system, or it may be totally blocked.

When the heart strains too much, the system breaks down in a heart attack, a stroke, or some other manifestation of heart disease.

Recently researchers have come up with another important factor in the cholesterol story. There are several different *kinds* of cholesterols. Most of these can be dismissed, but *two* are of great concern because they contradict each other.

LDLS AND HDLS—THE GOOD GUYS AND THE BAD GUYS

One of these cholesterols is a low-density lipoprotein (known popularly as "LDL"), and the other is a high-density lipoprotein (known popularly as "HDL").

To make it complicated, one of these is "good" and the other "bad," at least in the sense of helping reduce the accumulation of plaque on the inner surface of the arteries.

LDLs—the low-density lipoproteins—are the "bad guys." Tests have determined that they carry cholesterol to the body's cells, including those that line the walls of the coronary arteries, where major trouble can occur with plaque buildup. A high level of these LDLs in the body signals dangerous accumulations of deposits in the coronary arteries.

HDLs—the high-density lipoproteins—are the "good guys." Tests have determined that they help carry excess cholesterol *away* from the cells and back to the liver for processing or metabolizing for removal. A high level of HDLs in the bloodstream in relation to the level of LDLs usually means that the body is much less apt to be a prospect for coronary heart disease, and vice versa.

Dr. Basil Rifkind of the National Heart, Lung, and Blood Institute has said that, on the whole, the LDL count is a much better indicator of heart disease than the cholesterol count alone. In fact, he goes on to point out that the LDL count overrides such distinctions as gender and age differences in people, which were once thought to determine the individual's susceptibility to heart disease.[1]

How These HDLs and LDLs Act

These two cholesterol types act in special ways, almost as if they worked independently from the rest of the body.

For example, LDLs seem to be stimulated to appear in greater numbers—that is, in high counts of cholesterol—by cigarette smoking. Not only do the LDLs appear in greater numbers, but the HDLs tend to remove themselves from the scene. Thus cigarette smoking causes the "good guys" to depart and the "bad guys" to come flocking in to clog the arterial system!

TRIGLYCERIDES: THE OTHER BLOOD FATS

In addition to cholesterol, other lipids—blood fats—are present in the bloodstream. One of these is numbered as an important risk factor in heart disease—number four, as has been explained.

Called a triglyceride, this blood fat is a kind of cousin to cholesterol, but with a different chemical makeup. Nevertheless, triglycerides are similar to cholesterol blocks in that they are lipoproteins too, although they appear in plant life as well as in animal life.

Some triglycerides come from vegetable sources like corn oil or safflower oil. They are liquid at room temperature; they contain what is called "polyunsaturated fat." This is an important distinction, because of all fats ingested by the body, polyunsaturated fat is the "good" fat that does not induce the accumulation of cholesterol in the bloodstream as other fats do.

Other triglycerides often come from animal sources—bacon, butter, grease, and lard—and are solid at room temperature; they are rich in saturated fat. Obviously, this type of fat is "bad" for the body, inasmuch as it tends to induce the presence of cholesterol in the bloodstream.

What Triglycerides Do

In general, triglycerides are important to the body because they can either be deposited in fat cells or converted to immediate energy. The liver changes excess calories and foods like fatty acids, alcohol, and sugar into triglycerides for transportation in the bloodstream. Essentially, triglycerides are a storage form of fat in the body.

RISK FACTORS IN BLOOD CHOLESTEROL LEVELS

The most recent and generally accepted analysis of blood cholesterol levels has been determined by a panel of blue-ribbon experts representing twenty governments and private bodies. Its findings were first released October 19, 1987; those results are condensed and detailed here. The figures refer to milligrams of cholesterol in a deciliter of blood, expressed as "200 mg/dl," or 200 milligrams of cholesterol in a deciliter of blood.[2]

In general, there are three distinct levels of risk: a desirable level, a borderline level, and a dangerous level.

Desirable Level

A figure of 200 mg/dl or lower is a desirable cholesterol level in any plan of action you might adopt in fighting the accumulation of cholesterol in your arterial system. At this level, all you need to do is relax and continue the way you have been eating. However, your cholesterol levels must be checked every five years at least.

Borderline Level

These figures are called borderline figures. The borderline referred to is that between marginal risk and heavy risk. At this level, you should first of all modify your diet. The idea is to restrict total fat intake to 30 percent of your total intake in calories. You should also restrict the intake of saturated fat to 10 percent of your daily intake of calories. You should keep your dietary cholesterol intake to 300 milligrams per day. And you should check your blood levels at least once a year.

Dangerous Level

These figures are high. And high means dangerous. At this level, you must severely restrict your intake of fats. Your blood should be further analyzed for the presence of LDLs, the "bad" cholesterols. If, after six months, your LDL level remains excessive, you should try therapy with some kind of cholesterol-lowering drug, or a combination of them and a new diet.

TWO MORE RISK FACTORS: OVERWEIGHT AND CHOLESTEROL

The intake of fat tends to raise cholesterol and LDL concentrations in the blood; polyunsaturated fats tend to lower these concentrations. For example, by removing one gram of saturated fat from your diet, you lower your cholesterol level by approximately the same amount as is achieved by adding two grams of polyunsaturated fat to it!

Your triglyceride level is always increased by eating saturated fat, and it is decreased by eating polyunsaturated fat. The simplest way to lower your triglyceride level is to restrict your caloric intake. Obesity and the consumption of alcohol are two other main contributors to high levels of triglycerides in Americans.

NOTE: There are *no* values for blood levels of cholesterol or triglycerides that separate those at risk for coronary disease from those *not* at risk.

In parts of the world where the level of cholesterol is relatively low, less atherosclerosis occurs in the population at large and fewer deaths by coronary heart attack. In the U.S., the average cholesterol level for adults is 210 mg/dl, and this level rises with age. The higher the cholesterol level—particularly the level of LDLs—the greater the risk of dying of early heart attack.

HOW TO TELL WHO IS AT GREATEST RISK

In spite of any risk factor, every individual is different in his or her reaction to cholesterol in the bloodstream. Certain people may ingest far past the maximum "safe" level of cholesterol, and experience no noticeable accumulation. Others may ingest fairly "safe" amounts and yet suffer from unexpected accumulation.

Dr. Michael Brown of the University of Texas looks at the problem in this manner: "Some people are sensitive and some people are resistant [to sunburning]. The only problem is we can't just look at them and tell who is who."[3]

That is exactly the case with cholesterol buildup. There is no way to determine ahead of time exactly who will suffer most. With cholesterol, the best approach is to assume it will hurt you and cut down on your cholesterol intake. Also, be sure to have your cholesterol count monitored regularly.

RECOMMENDED CHOLESTEROL DIETS

Once you know your cholesterol level, you can either relax or begin an active dietary campaign. Proper diet is the best way to fight high cholesterol levels. Although certain drugs can be used to lower extremely high cholesterol counts and surgery can be performed for certain patients, the practical way to lower cholesterol levels is to begin a diet that has been prepared for this specific treatment.

The main target that is recommended by the American Heart Association: limiting your cholesterol intake to less than 300 milligrams per day and confining your intake of total fat to less than 30 percent of your total calories.[4]

The reduction of your intake of saturated fats and cholesterol may produce substantial decreases in blood cholesterol levels. However, if you continue to have a significantly elevated blood cholesterol level, you may want to consult a doctor about the use of some cholesterol-lowering drug.

STEP 1 AND STEP 2 DIETS

The blue-ribbon panel that devised the cholesterol levels already analyzed also came up with two types of anti-cholesterol diets: the Step 1 diet and the Step 2 diet.

The Step 1 diet is the milder diet; it involves cutting your caloric intake of fat to 30 percent. Your intake of saturated fat (animal fat) should be less than 10 percent of your entire caloric intake. You can accomplish this by limiting your meals to six ounces or less of lean meat, fish, or poultry (without skin). You should use only skim milk or other low-fat dairy products. Limit yourself to three egg yolks a week, and eat no butter at all. The main operative rule here is to *limit your intake of saturated fat.*

The Step 2 diet is the more severe and involves reducing your fat intake to 7 percent or less of your total calories. You limit yourself to one egg yolk a week and consume no saturated fat at all.

Mary Winston, the chief dietitian for the American Heart Association, points out: "People automatically think the diets can't taste good. That's simply not true."[5]

The Secret of One Egg Yolk

Standard dietary advice limits daily cholesterol consumption to the amount of cholesterol you get in one egg yolk. That's right! A whole egg provides 250 or more milligrams of cholesterol, and most of that comes from the yolk.

DIET AND EXERCISE—OR DIET OR EXERCISE?

By dieting, you can actually count your success by the numbers. If, for example, you lower your cholesterol level by one percentage point, lowering it from 215 to 213, you decrease the risk of heart disease by two percent. Your lowered risk is double the amount you take off. Thus, if you manage to cut down your cholesterol level five percentage points, you reduce your risk of heart disease by ten percent!

Dieting alone is actually not enough to bring down cholesterol levels, although it plays a major part in maintaining good health. Exercise is always a backup element in a good diet.

Eric Ravussin, a researcher at the National Institute of Diabetes and Digestive and Kidney Diseases in Phoenix, says that exercise keeps the muscle from turning into fat. Lack of exercise may not do so. The point is, the more fat a person's body carries in relation to muscle, the lower the resting metabolic rate. A low metabolic rate tends to allow fat to accumulate.[6]

In a study sponsored by the National Institute of Health to investigate cholesterol levels and blood pressure levels, Stanford's Center for Research and Disease Prevention found that a weight-loss program that combines diet *and* exercise is the best way to achieve the optimum physical and physiological benefits.

Dr. Peter Wood of Stanford compared test results of 155 healthy but overweight men, with those from three groups: an exercise-only group jogging ten miles a week; a diet-only group decreasing their caloric intake to 300 calories a day; and a control group with no variation in diet or exercise. The diet-only group lost sixteen pounds; the exercise group lost ten pounds. The percentage of body fat in both groups remained the same.

Wood determined from his studies that diet and exercise each reduced blood pressure levels and increased levels of high-density lipoprotein—HDLs, the "good" cholesterol—to help prevent heart disease. However, the final determination of the study was that the best way to better health is to combine both diet and exercise for a two-pronged attack.[7]

THE VALUE OF FISH IN A CHOLESTEROL DIET

Dr. David Blankenhorn, professor of medicine and director of atherosclerosis research at the University of Southern California Medical School, has recommended that patients suffering from cholesterol deposits should eat more fish.

"If you eat the flesh, such as salmon steak," he says, "you get the oil in the steak and [you] don't get much of the cholesterol [from the fish]." He notes that drinking cod liver oil might provide an overdose of vitamin D, and "Vitamin D is hard on the arteries as well as the kidneys." Even too much vitamin A can give you problems with your eyes and bones.[8]

Dr. Ruth Johnson, a U.S.C. nutritionist and heart disease researcher, advises people to consume six ounces of lean meat, fish, or poultry (without skin) a day, and at least twelve ounces of fish a week. Johnson believes that "moderation is still the very best practice" in any kind of dieting.[9]

She is echoed by Dr. Victor Herbert, an internationally known nutritionist: "There are no fast foods which are inherently bad or inherently good. No food is junk food in moderation, and any food is junk food without moderation."[10]

TYPICAL FOODS AND CHOLESTEROL COUNTS

Let's take a look at some foods you probably eat regularly just to see how much cholesterol they contain. First, watch out for the foods with too much cholesterol. You may or may not be surprised at the figures in this list:

- *A whole egg:* One egg will take up your entire daily quota—or almost a full day. One egg, containing 5.5 grams of fat, carries 250 milligrams of cholesterol!
- *Chicken liver:* One cup of chicken liver will take up two-and-a-half days of your entire cholesterol intake. That amount of chicken liver contains 4.4 grams of fat, with 746 milligrams of cholesterol.
- *Carrot cake:* A 3½-ounce slice of carrot cake contains 20.4 grams of fat and carries 30 milligrams of cholesterol.

• *Ice cream:* One cup of 16 percent ice cream contains 23.8 grams of fat and carries 84 milligrams of cholesterol.

Foods with a significant cholesterol content are listed in Table 3.1. Foods which have a lower cholesterol content and which you can eat without caution are listed in Table 3.2.

Table 3.1

High-Cholesterol Foods

Food	Fat Content	Cholesterol Content
Brownie, average	9.4 g	25 mg
Ground beef (27%) 3 ounces	16.9 g	86 mg
Butter, 1 T.	12.2 g	36 mg
Mayonnaise, 1 T.	11.0 g	5 mg
Ricotta cheese, 1/2 C. (13% fat)	16.1 g	63 mg
Yogurt, 1 T.	12.2 g	36 mg

Table 3.2

Low-Cholesterol Foods

Food	Fat Content	Cholesterol Content
Bread, whole wheat 1 slice	.8 g	-0-
Cottage cheese, 1/2 C. (1% fat)	1.6 g	5 mg
Egg white	-0-	-0-
Flatfish, 31/2 oz.	.8 g	66 mg
Margarine, 1 T.	12.0 g	-0-
Miracle Whip, 1 T.	7.0 g	5 mg
Sherbet, 1 C.	4.0 g	7 mg
Yogurt, frozen, 1 C.	3.0 g	10 mg
Yogurt, low-fat, 1 C.	3.4 g	14 mg

A SAMPLE ANTI-CHOLESTEROL MENU

Here's a sample approach to controlling cholesterol levels.

FOR BREAKFAST: Oatmeal, with sugar substitute, skim milk, English muffin, toasted

or

Whole wheat toast, 2 slices, with margarine and black raspberry "conserve"

Banana

FOR LUNCH: Sliced chicken breast in pita bread, with lettuce and dressing

Cold navy beans, cooked in tomato sauce, mustard, brown sugar substitute

Strawberries

FOR DINNER: Green salad, with non-oil dressing

Grilled salmon steak

Baked potato, with margarine

Broccoli

Apple-raisin pie, with crust baked with safflower oil

The foods listed in Appendix 1 are low in cholesterol and saturated fat and should be a part of the daily menus for your anti-cholesterol diet. The next section provides a wide variety of tasty recipes with low cholesterol counts.

Happy dining the anti-cholesterol way!

·4·

Anti-Stroke Diet

THE BATTLE AGAINST hypertension, or high blood pressure, is the second phase in the dietary campaign against heart disease. Hypertension is as common as grass. Although figures are inconclusive, since its very nature makes it a silent, invisible killer, estimates show that over sixty million Americans suffer from its effects at this very moment.

WHAT IS HYPERTENSION?

Actually, the term *hypertension* is a misnomer. What hypertension really means medically is high blood pressure. The dictionary definition is quite specific: "Hypertension: abnormally high blood pressure and especially arterial blood pressure; *also:* the systemic condition accompanying high blood pressure."

This disorder is the cause of many of humankind's most serious ailments, among them kidney failure and heart disease.

Hypertension is a condition of the circulatory system of the human body. To understand it, you must first be aware of how the circulatory system works and what its purpose is.

What the Circulatory System Does

The basic purpose of the circulation of the blood through the body is to carry a supply of oxygen and nutrients to all parts of the organism and to remove particles that are impure and detrimental to the body. Thus, blood acts as a bringer and a remover at all times. The stream of blood moves through the body via an intricate system of tiny pipelike tubes; this network is called the arterial system, with the arteries serving as the pipes.

The heart acts as a pump for the system to move the supply-laden blood through the arteries. Each beat of the heart pushes the blood through the vessels. The thickness of the arteries determines the amount of pressure to be exerted. Their diameter is regulated in turn by a system of chemicals and hormones that changes the opening of the vessels to whatever size the condition of the body demands.

When the body is in repose, for example, the arteries widen and the blood circulates slowly and easily throughout. When the body is involved in activity, the arteries narrow in order to force blood through the arteries more quickly.

In some situations, particularly with a buildup of cholesterol layers in the arteries, the blood has much less room to move than in a normal artery. With arteries that are permanently narrowed with cholesterol buildup, the heart is forced to push the same amount of blood to all parts of the body through a system that has become restricted by constriction. This buildup makes the heart work a great deal harder to perform its function.

Working in the High-Pressure Mode

If this strain on the heart becomes regular, it can eventually lead to heart failure, fatal heart attack, or stroke that paralyzes the body and impairs the kidneys as well.

In extreme cases, the entire human arterial system works at all times in a high-pressure mode. The arteries have stiffened into a set form and have lost the capacity to expand and contract with ease, if at all. When the arterial system loses its elasticity, the condition is called "high blood pressure," or "hypertension."

This condition is extremely dangerous to the entire body system. Hypertension overworks the heart, endangers the elasticity of the arteries, threatens the efficiency of the kidneys in eliminating waste from the system, and causes the brain to lack proper nourishment brought to it by fresh blood.

If blood pressure continues to remain high, life expectancy is reduced dramatically.

How to Measure Blood Pressure

Finding out blood pressure levels in a human being is quite simple. A device called a sphygmomanometer, composed of a rubber tube and a meter, is wrapped around the upper arm. The wrap is inflated with air to stop the flow of blood in the main arteries, and air is then released from the device.

The heart performs two actions to pump blood through the system. It squeezes to pump, and it relaxes to rest. These two actions combine to form the beat of the heart. The squeeze is called the systolic pressure; the rest is called the diastolic pressure. The sphygmomanometer measures both systolic pressure and diastolic pressure, with the measurements calibrated in millimeters of pressure.

Thus, the two figures noted in a blood-pressure reading are systolic and diastolic, in that order. The average reading of a normal healthy adult might be about 120/80, but these figures vary in different individuals. Age, condition of the arteries, and medical history all contribute to such a reading.

If the reading rises above 160/95, the pressure is considered too high. Figures of that size are considered hypertensive readings; the patient is considered to be suffering from high blood pressure.

THE TWO TYPES OF HYPERTENSION

Hypertension appears in two different forms: malignant hypertension and essential hypertension. Both types of the condition are considered dangerous.

Considering the most serious first, malignant hypertension is a situation in which high blood pressure has demonstrably affected the internal organs. That is, the internal organs have deteriorated to a noticeable degree because of the lack of adequate blood flow.

Essential hypertension is a more benign type of high blood pressure. It is usually diagnosed when no causative factors for the disease are apparent. Essential hypertension does not dramatically affect the internal organs.

WHAT HYPERTENSION CAN DO

High blood pressure can cause extensive and important internal damage to the human body. Some of these manifestations are as follows:

- *Heart attack.* The heart, pumping much harder than it was designed to, becomes enlarged and flabby. Clogged arteries may reduce the amount of blood it can pump. The attack occurs because the heart can no longer cope.
- *Stroke.* The brain, deprived of blood because of narrowed arter-

ies, may be afflicted by a stroke, which is a seizure caused by lack of proper oxygen to the blood vessels in the brain. Permanent damage to the entire body may result.
• *Kidney damage.* Narrowed and hardened arteries caused by hypertension prevent the kidneys from removing body wastes. These wastes build up in the blood and eventually poison the entire body mechanism.
• *Blindness.* The blood vessels in the eyes can be strained and swollen by the presence of hypertension. If the high pressure continues, blindness may eventually result when these vessels break down.
• *Arteriosclerosis.* (Not to be confused with *atherosclerosis.*) Untreated hypertension can cause a hardening and scarring of the outer walls of the arteries. This condition ("arterio" = of the arteries; "sclerosis" = hardening) causes the arteries to lose their flexibility and become otherwise ineffective.

WATCH OUT FOR THESE WARNING SIGNS!

Hypertension often announces itself in specific symptoms that should be viewed as a warning by nature of the onset of trouble. Most people are not aware of what they mean. Taken separately, each symptom does *not* signal hypertension; but a combination of them might. Here are some of the most significant indications:

• *Nosebleed.* A nosebleed with no apparent cause may signal the onset of hypertension.
• *Dizziness.* Dizziness when the diastolic pressure is about 110 may indicate the presence of hypertension.
• *Headache.* To be a true indication of hypertension, a headache must fulfill at least six basic requirements: it must be severe; it must be of recent origin; it must be localized in one specific part of the head; it must occur in early morning; it must be accompanied by nausea; vision must become progressively worse.
• *Breathlessness.*

THE CURE FOR HYPERTENSION

No simple and specific cure exists for hypertension. Through the years, many different factors have been found to be important contributors to this human condition, so the search simply continues to identify new individual causes.

In general, weight control, exercise, the amount and kinds of fats you ingest, and your intake of potassium, calcium, and magnesium are *all* believed to be a part of the total hypertension profile.

Ongoing studies continue to discover new evidence relating to hypertension either directly or indirectly. Weight control has always been one of the primary targets for the person suffering from high blood pressure. A recent study of people trying to lose weight shows that exercise can be beneficial in providing the proper psychological and physical attitudes for the dieter; thus, these findings about exercise definitely pertain to the person who is trying to reduce hypertension.

More News about the Fiber Foods

Other new findings also tend to enlarge the medical profession's knowledge of hypertension. One of the very latest involves not only the fight against cancer, but also the fight against high blood pressure. It focuses on dietary intake, particularly the ingestion of fiber foods.

In a general observation about good health, Dr. Martin H. Floch, a professor of medicine at Yale University, says: "Recommendations of many health organizations now form a consensus: The most effective diet for chronic disease prevention and treatment is liberal in complex carbohydrate and fiber and limited in fat."

Then he zeroes in on high blood pressure: "A high-fiber, low-fat diet may also help lower blood pressure and is associated with a low incidence of coronary heart disease; some believe it lowers the risk of colon cancer."[1]

Smoking and Hypertension

It cannot be repeated too often that smoking is one of the three major risk factors associated with hypertension. The rate of heart attacks and strokes in the middle-aged adult smoker is twice that of nonsmokers.

As already mentioned, smoking has been correlated with low levels of HDLs (the "good guys") in the bloodstream. Nicotine is poisonous and capable of permanently damaging the blood vessels, the heart, the kidneys, and the gastrointestinal tract. In addition to that, it is indirectly responsible for a rise in blood pressure levels.

Smoking also tends to depress the appetite, which can hopelessly confuse any dietary program you may wish to adopt as a regimen. Since one of the most efficacious ways to lower your blood pressure is to carry out a stringent program of diet and exercise, it is obvious that smoking will prevent a complete success on your part.

In fact, one irony of smoking is that it tends to depress your appetite—and, sure enough, when you *stop* smoking, you may possibly gain from fifteen to twenty pounds in the next several months!

Obesity and Hypertension

In spite of the fact that it is neither chic nor socially acceptable to be fat in today's society, many people *are* overweight. There are various *degrees* of overweight, from slightly plump to dangerously obese. To become a menace to bodily health, your weight must exceed 130 percent of the ideal average for your size and age.

From the beginning of medical interest in high blood pressure, obesity has been strongly associated with hypertension. For some reason, obese people have low levels of the "good" HDLs. Males can reduce their weight, decrease their LDL level, raise their HDL level, and improve the LDL to HDL ratios; women, unfortunately, cannot.

Obese people frequently do very little physical exercise. However, losing weight by physical exercise alone is simply not feasible. You must restrict your caloric intake *in conjunction with* a regimen of exercise.[2]

Stress and Hypertension

Although stress is number eight in our list of eight risk factors in heart disease, it is one of the genuinely important factors in hypertension. Your susceptibility to stress depends a great deal on the type of person you are.

Researchers have divided people into two basic types, labeling them Type A and Type B, in order to study the manner in which people react to problems or threats.

A Type A individual is a hard-driving, overly conscientious, time-haunted person who hardly ever takes a day off or goes on a vacation. A common slang term for a Type A is workaholic. No matter where the workaholic is, he or she usually reacts in an aggressive, almost explosive manner, immediately preparing to rush any challenge head-on, banners flying, gung ho to conquer.

A Type B individual is much the opposite: a low-key personality who likes to accept situations as they are and who is driven much less by deadlines and goals. This person reacts to a challenge in a rather relaxed manner, studies all alternatives, analyzes options, and *then* advances to neutralize or dismantle the challenge.

HYPERTENSION AND CHALLENGE

The psychological term *stress* refers to the manner in which an individual reacts to a challenge—particularly a physical or mental one that creates tension in one's persona. You respond to stress by an increase in the blood pressure level, hence the interest in stress reaction by the medical profession. You also experience an increase in the heart rate, the release of epinephrine (adrenaline) and norepinephrine (noradrenaline), and a rise in blood sugar.

The Type A individual is obviously susceptible to frequent rises in blood pressure—in short, to hypertension. Among the dangerous bodily reactions to stress for the Type A person is, of course, the high elevation of blood pressure. A way to reduce stress in a Type A individual is to encourage him or her to relax and enjoy life.

The way a person eats, incidentally, is a key to the way he or she reacts to environmental stress. If you bolt down your food, stand up while eating, smoke frantically while drinking coffee, or read a newspaper during your lunch, you probably are internalizing stress. This kind of behavior can also be a warning of possible elevated blood pressure and a tendency to hypertension.

HOW TO LOWER YOUR BLOOD PRESSURE THROUGH DIET

There are four basic ways in which you can use diet to help lower your blood pressure:

1. Lower your caloric intake.
2. Lower your fat intake.
3. Lower your sodium intake.
4. Lower your intake of food additives.

Let's consider these one by one. But first, it would be wise to make note of a generally acceptable *balance* of foodstuffs. As an overall plan for eating, try to stay within these parameters:

- Eat no more than 300 milligrams of cholesterol per day.
- Eat 50 percent of your calories as carbohydrates.
- Eat 20 percent of your calories as protein.
- Eat 30 percent of your calories as fat, with 1) less than 10 percent of fat from saturated fat; 2) up to 10 percent of fat from polyunsaturated fat; 3) the remaining fat from monounsaturated fat.

1. How to Lower Your Caloric Intake

A pound of fat equals about 3,500 calories. In order to lose two pounds a week, you must reduce your daily caloric intake by 1,000 calories.

Rationale: 1,000 calories × 7 days = 7,000 calories = 2 pounds per week.

First you should determine your present caloric intake. To do this, keep a food intake record for a week, tallying your calories with a food computer. At the end of the week, average your daily intake. Then make a corresponding food exchange.

Typical Food Exchanges

In the meat group, one *meat exchange* might be:

1/4 cup flaked, cubed, or chopped meat OR
1 ounce (30 gms) lean cooked meat

In the bread and cereal products group a *cereal exchange* might be:

1 slice bread OR
1/2 cup cooked macaroni OR
1/2 cup cooked cereal OR
1/4 cup sherbet OR
1/3 cup corn

In the dairy products group a *dairy exchange* might be:

1 cup skim milk OR
1 cup buttermilk (made with skim milk) OR
1/2 cup canned evaporated skim milk (undiluted) OR
1/3 cup nonfat dry milk product

You can also combine exchanges in one food:

1/2 cup creamed cottage cheese
=1 dairy exchange + 1 fat exchange

1 cup low-fat milk (11/2 to 2 percent butterfat)
=1 dairy exchange + 1 fat exchange

2. How to Lower Your Fat Intake

The body uses fat to transport fat-soluble vitamins, and to supply calories for energy when needed. The average American consumes about 40 percent of all calories as fat; about 15 percent are consumed as saturated fat, 7 percent as polyunsaturated fat, and the remaining 18 percent as monounsaturated fat. Most nutritionists consider this far too high a ratio of fat to total intake of food.

Actually, you should consume 30 percent of your total calories as fat:

1. Eat less than 10 percent as saturated fat.
2. Eat up to 10 percent as polyunsaturated fat.
3. Eat the remainder as monounsaturated fat.

Fat is present in many processed and fried foods. In baked goods fat may contribute half of the caloric content; in luncheon meats and sausages, approximately 75 percent of the total; and in fried foods, 40 percent to 60 percent.

WARNING: The amount and type of fat you eat plays an important role in the risk of heart disease. Thus:

1. Too much saturated fat tends to *increase* the level of cholesterol in the bloodstream.

2. Polyunsaturated fats help *reduce* cholesterol, but have the same caloric content as saturated fat.
3. Monounsaturated fats may lower cholesterol, but have the same caloric count as saturated fat.

Where These Fats Come From

Saturated fats occur in all animal foods and some vegetable products. Such fats are solid at room temperature. Most of the fat in butter, beef, cream, and whole milk is saturated fat, although a large amount of oleic acid—a monounsaturated fat—is also present. The few vegetable fats that contain saturated fats are coconut, palm, and palm kernel oil.

Polyunsaturated fats are liquid at room temperature. They are mostly of vegetable origin. However, fish fat is also a polyunsaturated fat.

Monounsaturated fats may lower blood cholesterol levels. These fats are found in olives, olive oil, peanuts, peanut oil, peanut butter, and avocados. Most nuts also contain monounsaturated fats.

Fats in foods: The fat in eggs is in the yolk: one egg yolk of 17 grams contains about 5.5 grams of fat. Fish has polyunsaturated fat, ranging from 1 to 20 percent. Chicken and turkey are low in fat, especially when the skin is removed. White poultry meat contains less fat than dark meat. Fat in oil is used in processing food such as salad dressings, sauces, cookies, candies, cheeses, frozen desserts, cereals, meat products, soups, and frozen vegetables in sauce.

3. How to Lower Your Sodium Intake

Sodium is required by the human body to regulate the amount of fluid and electrolytes in and out of the body cells. Proper regulation is needed to maintain the flow of blood to and from the heart. As Dr. Ralph E. Minear, a faculty member of the Harvard Medical School and an attending physician at Massachusetts General Hospital, has explained, sodium helps the arteriole system constrict the arteries to speed up the flow of blood.[3]

In the hypertension-prone individual, the presence of sodium may become a problem. Too much sodium in the system increases the fluid-holding capacity of the blood expanding the volume so that there is more blood present than needed. The situation created is conducive to raising the blood pressure level in the system.

In addition, sodium can also constrict the small blood vessels. By providing an excess of fluid in the blood and by constricting the arterioles (the small blood vessels), sodium thus provides a one-two punch to the heart. In the end, the heart is forced to work harder to push the expanded volume of blood through the constricted channels in the arterial system.

This added burden on the heart causes the most harm. The additional pressure can wind up forcing a breakdown or breakdowns in the system: heart attack, stroke, or kidney complications.

How Much Sodium Is Safe to Eat?

The National Research Council of the National Academy of Sciences recently determined that an "adequate and safe" sodium intake—one that would not lead to hypertension in the hypertension-prone—is about 1,100 to 3,300 milligrams of sodium a day for adults. Just to give you an idea of the size, that amount would be about 1.75 to 8.25 grams of table salt.

However, at the same time, a report reveals that the average sodium intake of a typical American is a great deal more than that. This average holds at about 8,000 to 12,000 milligrams of sodium a day—more than fifty times as much as the body *needs,* and about eight times the amount thought to be a safe level. Take note of these figures and remember them.

Lowering Your Sodium Intake

One practical way to cut down on your sodium intake is simply to put away your salt cellar in the cupboard and bring it out only for guests. Sodium is, of course, a chemical component (with chloride) in common table salt.

But acquaintance with a number of real sodium-intensive foods—common foods that you may not think of as containing large amounts of sodium—will help alert you to them as carriers of high amounts of sodium.

NOTE: Sodium is present in all drinking water, but in varying degrees. Utility-processed water for the home—the kind you draw when you turn on your tap—is usually high in material containing sodium, which is used as a purification agent. To avoid ingesting sodium in the water you drink, purchase bottled water with a low-sodium content.

Now for a list of foods with high sodium content. They are foods you should know about. If you can avoid these foods you can be confident that you are helping maintain a low level of sodium intake.

Foods High in Sodium Content

Anchovies	Meat canned or frozen in sauce
Bacon	Meat tenderizers
Baking powder	Monosodium glutamate (MSG)
Baking soda	Mustard
Barbecue sauce	Olives
Beef wieners	Pastrami
Bologna	Pepperoni
Bouillon cubes	Pickles
Buttermilk	Pizza
Canned soup	Pork wieners
Caviar	Pretzels
Celery salt	Salami
Cheese (except cottage)	Salted fish
Chili sauce	Salted meats
Chips	Salted nuts
Crackers	Salted popcorn
Cured ham	Sardines
Cured meat	Sausage
Diet soft drinks (over 2)	Smoked fish
Dried cod	Soy sauce
Frankfurters	Steak sauce
Garlic salt	Tomato juice
Herring	Turkey wieners
Ketchup	Vegetable juice
Luncheon meat	Worcestershire sauce

4. How to Lower Your Intake of Food Additives

"Few experts claim that salt is the sole cause of hypertension," the Harvard Medical School *Health Letter* stated in 1979. "Rather, they describe salt as an important contributing factor in the 10 to 20 percent of Americans who are genetically susceptible to high blood pressure. And for such persons, the hidden salt in processed food of the typical American diet is a real hazard."[4]

Believe it. It is not the sodium in table salt that is dangerous; *that* is a visible entity. But for centuries sodium—as sodium chloride (table salt)—has been used not only in cooking, but in food-processing generally. Even today it is used in the curing of fish and meat. Sodium forms brine for olives, sauerkraut, and pickles. Sodium enhances the leavening of bread in baking. Sodium is used as a food intensifier to make natural flavor more flavorful.

Sodium is used to make cheese turn out the way the cheesemaker wants, because sodium controls fermentation in cheese and in many other products. Most important, in its preservative stance, sodium inhibits the growth of harmful bacteria in bread, bacon, and sausage.

As has been noted, in many cases sodium is *hidden* in food processing. For example, it occurs in the form of disodium phosphate in all kinds of "instant" cooking preparations. Most people really do not realize what the suggested 1,100 to 3,300 milligrams of sodium actually *look like* in foodstuffs. One serving of canned chicken noodle soup—say, one cup—supplies at least half a day's allowance of sodium! Other processed foods—cheese, tomato juice, ice cream—contain significant quantities of sodium that remain out of sight to the consumer.

KNOW YOUR FOOD ADDITIVES

One good way to find out how much sodium is contained in food additives is to remember how the commercially packaged foods you buy are actually processed. Then, by studying the labels, you can analyze the ingredients that contain sodium—since the word is usually linked with some other chemical term or terms.

For example, here is a good check list of food additives, with an explanation of the kinds of foods the particularly high-sodium additive is used for:

- *Brine.* This combination of salt and water is used to process corned beef, sauerkraut, and pickles—among other products.
- *Disodium phosphate.* This processing agent is used in preparing quick-cook cereals, as well as all kinds of cheeses.
- *Monosodium glutamate (MSG).* This chemical is used as a seasoning to intensify flavor in home food as well as restaurant food, and occurs as well in the preparation of many frozen foods.
- *Sodium alginate.* This preparation is used in the making of ice cream and chocolate milk to give it smoothness of texture.
- *Sodium benzoate.* This is a preservative used to prepare sauces, condiments, and commercial salad dressings.

- *Sodium hydroxide.* This preservative is used in the processing of fruits, hominy, and olives in order to soften and loosen the skins.
- *Sodium propionate.* This chemical inhibits the growth of bacteria in cheese and in baked goods.
- *Sodium sulfite.* This is a preservative used in some dried fruits and foods with artificial coloring, like maraschino cherries.

In Chapter 1 we mentioned that we were going to provide a synthesis of the medical knowledge about nutrition and health to combat cancer, stroke, and heart disease. One aspect we've yet to consider is exercise and the ways it can reduce your susceptibility to these three diseases. We'll consider that in the next chapter.

·5·

Exercise and Your Health

DESPITE ALL THE sweating and the huffing and puffing, we all know that exercise makes us feel better. Maybe not while our muscles are burning, but later on, the benefits become obvious. We can feel our mental and physical energy increase. We tend to work more effectively, maintaining better concentration as well.

Inside our bodies, where we can't see what's happening, subtle changes are occurring. Exercise can actually change our body's chemistry.

The mechanism by which exercise works is still being explored, but certain things have been verified. As we exercise aerobically (more on this later), the exercising muscles develop a greater capacity to remove and use oxygen from the blood. This change is linked to an increase in the energy-producing components of the muscle cells, including some enzymes. This, in turn, results in an increased work capacity for your muscles. In other words, the more you exercise the more you *can* exercise.

Have you ever noticed how you get a second wind after a long workout? That's the phenomenon of aerobic exercise. Did you ever exercise for several weeks and notice that the exercise has become much easier since you first started? That's it too.

Not only does this occur for the body as a whole, but also for that one special muscle, your heart. Because of its increased strength and efficiency, your now-stronger heart needs to pump fewer times to supply the same amount of blood. This newly exercised heart clearly operates under less stressful conditions, and that's a great change.

There's a positive chemical change here too. Blood levels of heart-stimulating hormones (such as adrenalin) are lower after exercising, and this results in less stressful heart action also.

While research in this area is still relatively new, scientists have demonstrated that certain kinds of exercise not only strengthen the heart, but also can increase the amount of high-density lipoprotein (HDL), commonly called "good cholesterol." Because exercise decreases body fat, fit people also see a subsequent decrease in chemical compounds such as low-density lipoprotein (LDL), the so-called "bad cholesterol." These changes in cholesterol tend to decrease blood clotting and, along with that, reduce the chance of stroke and heart attack.

In case you find all this hard to believe, the hard data is rather impressive.

THE MEDICAL FACTS ABOUT EXERCISE

The Centers for Disease Control in Atlanta conducted a two-year analysis of research projects that studied exercise and heart disease. Their extensive data, released in 1988, showed a significant relationship between the lack of exercise and coronary heart disease.

The CDC found that people with the lowest levels of physical activity had a risk of heart disease almost two times greater than those at the highest physical activity levels.

Dr. Carl Caspersen, a CDC researcher, said, "The results indicate that physical inactivity raises your risk of heart disease. In general, most studies have seemed to indicate that, but no one has looked at it quite as carefully as we did."

Another study, reported in 1987 by researchers at the University of Minnesota, showed that men who regularly exercised either moderately or intensely experienced a 37 percent lower adjusted risk of cardiac death than did sedentary men. In addition, the exercisers showed a 30 percent lower risk of overall mortality than the nonexercisers.

This long-term study included twelve thousand participants and seven years of follow-up studies. The average man exercised thirty-two minutes a day. Those who reported very high levels of exercise also reduced their risk of heart disease. However, it wasn't clear whether additional exercise gave greater protection or not.

Dr. Arthur Leon, who headed the study, said, "the principal mechanism may be the improved physical fitness of the heart. . . . Additional potential benefits of regular physical activity included helping to maintain body weight, [helping one stop] cigarette smoking, increasing high-density lipoprotein cholesterol levels, lowering of blood pressure levels and improv[ing] glucose insulin dynamics."

While very few experts dispute the positive effects of exercise, what *is* up for debate—and where most of the research now is centered—is how much exercise and what kind; does it work for those who've already had heart disease; and is it beneficial for older people or those who've never exercised before?

WHAT KIND OF EXERCISE IS BEST?

Fitness gurus divide exercise into two kinds: anaerobic (or isometric) and aerobic (or isotonic). *Anaerobic* (meaning "without oxygen") exercise includes activities such as sprinting and weight-lifting. While they may build muscle tone and strength, they offer little to strengthen the cardiovascular system. During these exercises, your body tends to use more oxygen than it takes in. How do you know if you're doing an anaerobic exercise? Easy—after you're done, you feel as if you're about to collapse.

Moreover, research has shown that exercises such as weight-lifting can *increase* blood pressure, especially in unfit people and may actually *decrease* HDL (good cholesterol) levels.

Except for earning that hard-muscled stomach that you crave so much (and perhaps the ability to twist off stubborn jar caps without using that flat rubber pancake gizmo), anaerobic exercise is almost useless.

Aerobic (meaning "with oxygen") exercise, however, is a different story. Aerobic activities include jogging, bicycling, swimming, brisk walking, skating, and cross-country skiing. During these activities your body requires a relatively modest amount of oxygen. Unlike anaerobic exercises, once you're in shape you can do these activities for a prolonged amount of time, sometimes for hours, without becoming exhausted. Your breathing becomes more regular and you reach a point where you're not really out of breath, the much sought after "second wind."

After you've done it regularly, aerobic exercise actually increases your overall energy levels as it builds a healthier cardio-vascular system. Also, aerobic exercise burns calories and tends to lower your weight: another desirable benefit. There's almost nothing bad to say about aerobic exercise.

A LITTLE IS BETTER THAN NONE

Okay, so you're ready to do some aerobic exercise. How long should you exercise? Does a person who exercises forty minutes a day get double the results of someone who exercises only twenty minutes? Or does the benefit fall off after a certain time period? Is walking slowly for only a few minutes a day better than not walking at all?

Although all the results aren't in, some research indicates that *any* kind of exercise is better for you than *no* exercise at all. While many people think that, in order to become healthier, you must exercise rigorously, like running a marathon, that's not necessarily true.

One of the most dramatic findings came from the Institute for Aerobic Research in Dallas in 1990. An eight-year study of 10,244 men and 3,120 women—all in good health when the survey began—showed the premature death rate (per 10,000) was 18.6 for the fittest men, 27.1 for men who exercised only moderately, and 64 for sedentary men. The numbers for the women were similar. The main point was that any kind of exercise, no matter how moderate, was beneficial.

On the other side, recent research seems to bolster the thought that although too much exercise won't harm you (except for perhaps a strained muscle once in a while) you may reach a point where cardiovascular benefits drop off.

HOW DO I KNOW IF I'M WORKING HARD ENOUGH?

Generally, doctors recommend that you exercise for at least thirty minutes, three to four times a week. During each session you should exercise hard enough to make your heart beat at a level within your "target zone."

To determine your target zone, you must first calculate your maximum heart rate. Do that by subtracting your age from the number 220. Your target zone, then, will be 60 to 75 percent of your maximum heart rate.

Take, for example, a thirty-five-year-old man. His maximum attainable heart rate is: $220 - 35 = 185$. His target zone is then 60 to 75 percent of 185, or 111 to 139 beats per minute.

It's best for sedentary people to check with their doctors before beginning any exercise program. Your physician may also recommend a stress test before you begin. If your heart or lungs are damaged and you don't know it, trying to attain your target zone could be dangerous.

HOW LONG SHOULD I EXERCISE?

If you ask ten different experts how long to exercise, you'll get ten different answers. Therefore, the following times are average and not to be taken as absolute amounts. Only your doctor or physical fitness trainer can determine your exact needs and capacities.

Any exercise session should begin with a warm-up period of five or ten minutes. Check your pulse before you begin and then again after you've warmed up with easy stretches and gentle movements.

The easiest place to check your pulse is on the arteries in your wrist or neck. Use your index finger and middle finger to feel it. Don't use your thumb; it has a pulse of its own and may confuse you.

Most people check their pulse for ten seconds and multiply the number by six to get beats per minute. Your pulse should be very much lower than your target zone during warm-up.

After you've warmed up, slowly step up the pace of your exercise. After about five minutes, check your pulse again to see if you've reached your target zone. If you haven't reached it, increase your pace a little more. If you've exceeded your target range, slow down.

You want to stay within your target range for about twenty minutes or so.

After that, you must cool down. Let your body slow down and relax gradually. Slow down your pace for five to ten minutes. When you check your pulse it should be lower than your target range. If not, you're still going too fast.

Keep in mind that your recommended target zone may still be too severe an exercise for you. A good indication that you're going too fast is if it takes longer than fifteen minutes for your pulse to reach its normal pace after exercising. Other signs of a too intense workout are difficulty breathing, feeling dizzy or faint, or prolonged weariness.

After a few weeks of exercise, you'll find that it will take more and more activity to reach your target zone. That's a good sign. It means that your heart is getting stronger.

Now that you know about operating in your target zone, you should also know that a growing number of doctors believe it's a dumb idea to stay at the high end. Studies suggest that operating steadily in the 60 percent area yields significant benefits. One study, performed by the Stanford University School of Medicine, compared three groups of twenty-five middle-aged subjects over a twelve-week period. The first group consisted of those who didn't exercise; the second group was composed of those who exercised at 60 percent of their target zone; the last group exercised at high intensity, or 75 percent of their target zone.

The lower group achieved a 10 percent improvement in aerobic capacity, while those in the 75 percent range improved 14 percent. Not a great difference, is it?

The Stanford study also distinguished between the *health* benefits of exercise, such as better cholesterol levels, and the *fitness* benefits of exercise, such as greater stamina. Some scientists believe that health benefits can be achieved with lower levels of exercise, and only people who also want the fitness benefits need to believe in T-shirts that tout "no strain, no gain."

LISTEN TO YOUR BODY

There are always dangers involved in rigorous exercise, not only to the heart but to the rest of your body. For example, runners sometimes experience pain in their shins and knees. Swimmers may feel leg cramps or pains in their sides. If you experience any pain or discomfort beyond a minor stretched muscle (especially if you've never been very active before) see your physician. Be aware of abnormal heart rhythms, palpitations, dizziness, headache, nausea, vomiting, or prolonged muscle pain. It could indicate a serious problem.

Because the target zone numbers can vary so much from person to person, some trainers suggest doing away with it altogether and replacing it with something called the "Borg Scale of Perceived Exertion."

The Borg scale was developed by Swedish fitness expert Gunnar Borg and tracks exercise on a scale of six to twenty. Six is very, very light exertion while twenty is very, very heavy. Exercisers match their perception with the scale. This deemphasis on the heart rate number places less pressure on people to reach a specific goal and more importance on how they feel about their personal accomplishments. This method, say some trainers, encourages more people to exercise and keep at it longer. They contend that people are more likely to exercise if they see it as fun and not as a goal that must be met.

The Borg scale is especially suited to overweight and out-of-shape people who might be discouraged if they can't exercise in their target zone for twenty minutes.

Whether you adhere to the target zone method, the Borg scale, or any other method, the key is to exercise regularly. The next question, of course, is what kind of exercise.

HOW TO CHOOSE THE BEST EXERCISE FOR YOU

Besides diet, many other components of your lifestyle can reduce the risk of heart disease and cancer. Although this is a nutrition book, if you are going to be aggressive about preventing disease, you should keep these activities in mind. Exercise is the first nondiet activity you should pursue. Research shows that exercise can reduce your chance of heart attack and stroke, lower cholesterol, and improve your resistance to infection. The combined effects of exercise and diet are greater than one or the other alone. If you want your diet to be the most effective, exercise along with it.

Exercise doesn't necessarily mean running five miles or swimming a mile a day (although those aren't bad ideas); exercise means becoming more active than you are now, and on a regular basis. If you take a mile-long bus trip to work, walk instead. If you drive three miles to work in a car, switch to a bicycle. If your office is on the seventh floor, skip the elevator and take the stairs. Whatever you choose, exercise doesn't have to be difficult. Buy a stationary bicycle and place it in front of your television; you can watch the news and improve your health at the same time. Square dancing is a terrific exercise too.

If you've not had time to participate in a sport for decades, find time now. Consult your doctor before starting any exercise program if you have not been active for the past few years. The Committee on Exercise of the American Heart Association says: "We do *not* consider it justifiable to advocate widespread adoption of vigorous exercise programs purely on the ground that exercise alone will prevent heart disease." Don't jump the gun: Be sure you have a doctor's approval before you begin again.

Deciding which aerobic exercise you want to use will depend upon whether you want to be inside or outside, whether you want to use equipment, and which activity appeals to you. Let's look at the pros and cons of each kind of exercise.

Walking

Walking is the simplest, most accessible, and least likely to cause injury of all aerobic activities. Unless the weather is particularly severe, you can usually do it all year long. In many areas, people walk in enclosed shopping malls when it's very hot or cold outside. Some malls even open their doors an hour earlier than the stores, just for walkers.

As for equipment, walking requires only a pair of good shoes. Unless you have foot problems, any kind of supportive shoe is fine.

Jogging

Jogging requires a little more planning than walking. Most important is that you buy proper footwear. Entire books have been written about how to buy jogging shoes, but if you don't want to read them, you probably can get all the information you need at a reputable athletic footwear store.

Jogging usually produces better fitness in the same amount of time as walking because the body must work harder.

Although jogging used to be all the rage, it's fallen out of favor because of injuries you can sustain if you're not in good shape or if you're not careful. For instance, sports medicine doctors see many runners with "shin splints," an injury caused by constant shock to the leg. Sometimes it's caused by shoes without the proper cushioning. Sometimes it is caused by running too heavily or for too long. It's not uncommon for people to reach the so-called "runner's high" where, buoyed by a mental euphoria, they continue beyond their physical limits and unknowingly hurt themselves.

Swimming

Swimming is considered one of the best aerobic workouts, because it works the major muscle groups of the upper and lower body, as well as the cardiovascular system. The bonus in swimming is that it's a very low-impact activity—it's almost impossible to injure yourself unless you hit your head on the pool's edge. The main drawback to swimming is inconvenience. You must be able to get to a large-sized pool on a regular basis.

Bicycling

Although not as vibration-free as swimming, bicycling is relatively easy on your joints. Other than its obvious aerobic component, bicycling is fun and allows you to be outside in the fresh air and sunshine. One of the main complaints about exercise is that it's boring. Biking is rarely tedious or routine, especially in a big city complete with buses, taxis, and other bikers.

Stationary Cycling

This gives you all the physical benefits of regular biking without the other concerns of weather and traffic. And the new types of stationary bikes even have gadgets that simulate hills and straightaways. This not only allows you to vary your workout, but helps alleviate the boredom of staying in one place.

Jumping Rope

The exercise of prizefighters, this is one of the hardest types of aerobic exercises to sustain. It's really for those who have brought their bodies up to a high fitness level. One of the main benefits is that it builds good coordination. It's rather unforgiving, however, and unlike some other aerobic exercises, you can't let your mind wander too far. Not recommended for klutzes.

Skating

This is an excellent exercise and also a great social opportunity. Ice skating, of course, used to be available only in the winter, but with indoor rinks, you can "beat the heat" during the summer too. Roller skating, of course, is accessible all year. Like biking, it can be dangerous due to road obstacles, but it's never the same each time. Good balance and coordination are necessary.

Cross-Country Skiing

This requires a high degree of fitness, but it can be very rewarding because of the beautiful terrain you can travel through. The only thing to be aware of is extreme cold weather. It's important not to sweat and have that perspiration freeze. Warm-up exercises, although important for all aerobic activities, are critically important for cross-country skiing because low temperatures can tighten and tense your muscles.

Aerobic Dancing

This is what most people simply call "aerobic exercise." It's moving your arms and legs in place to music. The best part of it is, like walking, your only investment is in a good pair of shoes—and of course the latest, most expensive aerobic outfit!

Despite its simplicity, the medical consensus about aerobics has changed over the years. Now many experts suggest "low impact" aerobics, which is designed to lessen the shock or impact on your legs and arms. Its primary emphasis is on controlling your motion. This not only reduces injury, but makes the movements more graceful.

WARMING UP AND COOLING DOWN

No matter which exercise you choose, you must always preface it with a warm-up period and end with a cool-down period. Both *must* be included in your program. Warming up helps raise your heart rate slowly, thus avoiding injury to your cardiovascular system. Starting (or finishing) too fast can cause an irregular heartbeat and make you feel out of breath before you've gone very far.

Second, unless you warm and stretch your muscles you could sustain a sprain or tear. By allowing yourself a slow start, basically "getting the blood pumping," your muscles and the rest of your body are assured of an adequate and gently increasing supply of blood, oxygen, and nutrients. And slowing down gradually keeps your blood flowing more evenly, preventing muscle stiffness.

A typical program consists of five or ten minutes of stretching exercises and slow movements. The following exercises can be used for warm-ups and cool-downs, and it's important to do them slowly and deliberately. Perform each movement for one to two minutes. The order in which you do them isn't crucial; correct form is. Never bounce or strain.

1. *Sit-ups:* Lie on your back with your arms folded flat across your chest. Bend your knees so that your feet are squarely on the ground. By contracting your abdominal muscles, lift your head and shoulders off the ground. Your arms should touch your legs just above the knees. Don't strain to go all the way. Go as far as you can without hurting yourself. As you progress, you'll be able to do them fully.

2. *Modified Sit-ups:* If regular sit-ups are too difficult for you at first, try this version. Lie on your back, palms down with your knees slightly bent. Raise your head slightly as if you were looking over your chest, and hold for a few seconds. Repeat. Be sure you contract your stomach muscles (not your neck) to perform this movement.

3. *Reach and Bend:* Stand straight, your feet about shoulder-width apart. Extend your hands above your head as far as you can without lifting your feet off the floor. Now, bend forward at the waist and touch the floor or as far as you can go. Bend your knees slightly. Repeat slowly, five times on each side.

4. *Pelvic Thrust:* Lie flat on your back with your arms relaxed at your sides. Push the curve of your lower back against the floor. You'll be pulling in your stomach muscles as you do it. Hold, then repeat.

5. *Knee Kiss:* Lie flat on your back and pull one knee to your face by clasping it with your locked hands. Don't worry if you can't pull it all the way up. Hold. Repeat with each leg separately.

6. *Heel Cord Stretcher:* Place your palms flat on a wall about three feet in front of you. Keep your feet on the floor and your back straight as you slowly bend your arms and move closer to the wall. Hold. Repeat.

7. *Thigh Stretch:* Lie on your side with both legs straight. Grab your right ankle with your right hand and pull back until your heel touches your buttock. Hold. Repeat several times, then turn over and do the other leg.

8. *Leg Stretch:* Sit with your legs slightly spread apart. Put your right hand on your inner right thigh for support while you grab the inside of your left foot with your left hand. Keep your back straight

as you slowly straighten your leg and lift it to about a forty-five-degree angle. Hold. Repeat with the other leg.

9. *Overhead Arm Stretch:* Stand two to three feet from a wall. With the wall to your left side, place your left palm flat on the wall. Bend sideways at the waist as you lift your right arm past your ear and over your head. Hold and repeat with the other arm.

ARE YOU EVER TOO OLD TO EXERCISE?

The answer is an emphatic *NO.* Research has shown that elderly people, even those who have never exercised, can benefit by beginning a program immediately.

At about age thirty our bodies begin to show signs of normal wear and tear. Muscle strength declines, flexibility decreases, our coordination suffers, and we don't heal as quickly. Organs don't function as efficiently as they did before.

These are all indications of normal aging. However, researchers believe that beginning an exercise program not only increases your capacity to work, but also increases flexibility, strength, coordination, and other normally diminishing characteristics.

As with younger people, the elderly can also expect to see other beneficial effects of exercise such as lower blood pressure, improved cholesterol levels, and weight loss.

Older people, obviously, must be more careful about beginning an exercise regimen. A medical check-up is mandatory. So is a highly controlled, low-impact program such as walking or stationary bicycle riding.

If the target zone method is used to measure the level of exercise, older participants should aim for the lower end, around 60 percent of the maximum attainable heart rate. Also, because their muscles are less flexible, warm-ups become even more important for preventing stiffness and injury.

Elderly people should also keep their exercise time within the low target zone—about ten or fifteen minutes—and should remain at that level many more weeks than young people before moving on.

It's important to drink water before and after you exercise. Older people don't usually register thirst as soon as young people. This is especially important in warmer climates.

EXERCISE AND HEART ATTACK

Medical advice on exercise for those who have experienced heart attacks or strokes has completely reversed in recent years. Doctors used to tell patients to rest extensively; they now recommend exercise as a key ingredient for recovery from cardiovascular disease. Even as soon as a few weeks after a heart attack, patients are urged to start an exercise program. Studies have shown that inactivity after a heart attack can increase the risk of complications, such as blood clots and angina. Exercise can often build the heart to a condition better than before the attack.

Stress and Your Heart

As with exercise, stress plays a part in how healthy your heart is. Stress—anxiety, a fast-paced environment, too little free time, feeling guilty about doing nothing, always thinking about work, lack of self-confidence—will take a toll on your body. Real physiological changes—increased blood pressure and pulse rate, increased adrenalin production—occur in people who are under stress. Over time, these changes have adverse effects. Heart attacks occur more frequently in people who work (or live) in stress-inducing environments. Stress puts strain on your hormonal and nervous systems—strain that, in lay terms, "wears out the parts faster."

While you can't always change your environment (especially where you work), you can take steps to curtail the amount of stress you endure. There are numerous books available on how to minimize the stress in your life. Take time to enjoy relaxing activities, take vacations, get enough sleep, pursue those hobbies you haven't made time for lately, spend time with the people you love. And, of course, exercise.

EXERCISE AND CANCER

While the relationship between exercise and heart disease is well established, the association between exercise and cancer is still relatively new ground.

It's generally accepted that exercise relieves stress and that stress can be a factor in some cancers. However, it's also possible that lower cholesterol levels—a benefit of exercise—can actually increase your risk of cancer.

For instance, the now famous Framingham (Mass.) heart study, begun in 1948 and still ongoing, showed that the higher the male patients' cholesterol, the lower their cancer risk!

On the other hand, a study in Sweden showed just the opposite: Men with high cholesterol levels were 60 percent more likely to have colon and rectal cancer than those with lower levels.

Yet another study out of the Kaiser Permanent Medical Care Program in Oakland, California, showed no relationship at all between cholesterol and cancer. Who knows what to believe? Clearly, more research needs to be done on the link between cancer and cholesterol before doctors can agree.

Aside from the cholesterol connection, researchers have recently begun to look at other chemical compounds that may play a role in cancer. One study, made public in 1990, looked at heart, liver, and muscle tissues from rats that were trained to exercise regularly. Scientists at the University of Michigan discovered that the rats showed higher than normal levels of myoglobin and coenzyme Q, compounds that are normally present in cells and increase with exercise. These two compounds provide resistance to damage by chemically unstable molecules associated with cancer-causing agents. Whether these findings will hold true in humans hasn't yet been established.

A study in 1988 appears to agree with these preliminary results. Harvard biologist Rose Frisch examined more than five thousand athletic women and discovered that their reported incidence of breast and uterine cancer was half that of other women. Frisch saw an interesting chemical interplay here. She found that the active women produced a less potent form of estrogen than women who didn't exercise. Tumors that relied on that hormone didn't develop as easily.

EXERCISE AND STROKE

Kelley Brownell of the University of Pennsylvania School of Medicine refers to a study emphasizing exercise, attitudes, social support, and nutrition in weight loss, and points out that people who want to lose weight should find a good program that emphasizes permanent lifestyle changes over quick weight loss. He says that slow and safe weight loss, without the aid of pills, and without gimmicks like miracle foods, does the most good.

Identifying exercise as one of the most beneficial of all these elements in weight loss, Brownell explains: "It's a symbol that you're doing something positive."[1]

Anxiety and stress have also figured prominently in the medical profession's attempts to control hypertension. In a recent study including both world-class marathon runners and "fitness runners" logging in about twenty miles a week, David C. Nieman of the School of Health at Loma Linda University in California has discovered that exercise itself tends to relieve both anxiety and stress.

"I see increasing evidence that physical activity does help alleviate some of the symptoms associated with depression and anxiety and stress," Nieman says.[2]

In a similar study of women marathoners, William P. Morgan, professor of physical education and director of the Sports Psychology Laboratory at the University of Wisconsin, notes: "There is a tendency for runners and all athletes to be less depressed, and lower in anxiety and tension."[3]

Because of the great interest in exercise and disease, we can expect researchers to continue their experiments, one day perhaps discovering the exact association between the two. Whether that day actually comes or not, it's clear enough now that exercise is beneficial to our health, fitness, and general well-being. Exercise and a healthy diet should be partners in any total lifestyle.

·6·

The Three-in-One Concept

BY NOW THE question "What in the world can I eat?" has been answered. Cabbage. Fish. Oats. Kale. As you reviewed the list, another question probably surfaced in your mind: "Do I really *want* to eat what I *can* eat?" You are not happy about waving goodbye to the smell of bacon wafting up the stairs on a Sunday morning. Or that plate of Mom's spaghetti. Or that roast beef dinner with plenty of mashed potatoes and gravy, traditionally touted as "a man's dinner." Or that heaping dish of homemade ice cream. You may be wondering if, in fact, it's really worth avoiding these three major diseases.

Yes, it is. The healthful foods in the three-in-one diet can be just as delicious as those old favorites if you know how to prepare the new dishes properly. In Chapters 2, 3, and 4 of this book, we looked at each of these dreaded diseases individually, giving you general guidelines as to how to decrease your susceptibility to them. We warned you to beware of pesticides on produce, and suggested several alternatives—organic produce from the grocery store or your local farmers' market, and also washing hard-skinned produce in a mildly soapy solution—as a way to reduce your susceptibility to the poisons in pesticides, which can cause cancer and numerous other problems.

Instead of leaving you with just these general rules for the three individual diseases, chef Heather Harney has taken this research and used it to develop recipes for meals that will truly be "three-in-one," reducing your susceptibility to all three diseases at one time. Part Two of this book will present those recipes, and

Heather will introduce each recipe in that section with its particular benefits, so you will know the advantages of each dish.

Heather used three guidelines in developing her three-in-one recipes: the four factors that reduce your susceptibility to all three diseases, the two factors that have the double benefit of reducing your susceptibility to two of these diseases, and the three important factors in reducing your susceptibility to cancer, which could not be overlooked. And for those who are sensitive to alcohol, the recipes have been developed with nonalcoholic wines. You are free, of course, to make substitutions.

FOUR FACTORS THAT MAKE THREE-IN-ONE RECIPES POSSIBLE

You may have noticed that four factors were mentioned in each of the individual chapters on cancer, heart attack, and stroke. You can reduce your susceptibility to all three diseases if you:

1. Reduce your fat intake.
2. Eat more high fiber foods.
3. Consume less salt.
4. Eat foods with fewer additives and artificial-sounding ingredients.

Heather used these four factors as the benchmarks of the recipes she developed. Let's look at each one of them.

1. Reduce Your Fat Intake

If we were to inventory refrigerators across the United States, we'd find an incredibly rich assortment of condiments, such as mayonnaise, and salad dressings rich in creamy sauces and blue cheese. We'd also find a generous supply of milk, eggs, butter, sour cream, and cheeses such as cheddar, Swiss, and jack.

Yet in order to reduce our susceptibility to these three diseases we need to reduce the amount of eggs, butter, margarine, mayonnaise, milk, and cheese in our diets. How discouraging when we've been raised to enjoy milkshakes, typically American dishes like macaroni and cheese, which are high in fat, and snacks like pizza.

The good news is: You don't have to give up milkshakes and pizza and hamburgers altogether. Coffee ice cream lovers will find a recipe for a Coffee Milkshake (p. 201), which is nearly nonfat, in Part Two. Heather has also included some very creative recipes for pizza: White Pizza with Rosemary (p. 227), which uses ricotta cheese (a soft cheese that's low in fat, sodium, and calories), Vegetarian Pizza (p. 226), which is fairly low in fat (5.4 grams per serving), and a recipe for Pizza Dough (p. 93), which omits the salt and is higher in nutrition than most pizza because it uses wheat germ. There is even a recipe for Special Hamburgers (p. 190), which uses a low-fat cut of beef and is seasoned with sweet red pepper, garlic, cayenne pepper, and no-salt-added Dijon mustard instead of a lot of salty condiments. Heather suggests that you try Special Hamburgers with Peppered Yam Fries (p. 136), her alternative to French fries.

The recipes in this book propose a new source of sauces and salad dressings, which still provide some of the very familiar flavors of Barbecue Sauce (p. 154), Ketchup, (p. 154), and assorted vinaigrettes (pp. 173, 174). Yet you won't have to spend hours standing over a hot stove manufacturing an entire assortment of new sauces and salad dressings. Many of the recipes are basic and can be used in a number of ways. For instance, most of the sauces are excellent accompaniments to a variety of meats and fishes. Many of them can also be used as dips. Herbed Garlic Dressing (p. 169), Lemon Tarragon Dressing (p. 170), and Sesame Dip (p. 231), for instance, can be used as light cheese spreads for toasted bread, as flavored mayonnaises for sandwiches, and as great dips to replace the sour cream variety. These dressings are just as delicious as that creamy sour cream and garlic dressing— and that onion soup dip—you've come to love so much. And Heather has other replacements for that fat ogre, sour cream. Thickest Yogurt (p. 88) can replace sour cream on potatoes and in Mexican dishes. It can also replace the mayonnaise in luncheon salads. It can be sweetened and used as a garnish for fruit desserts and as a base for rich desserts, like Mocha Almond Pudding (p. 212). Heather suggests that you make one large batch of Thickest Yogurt, and then you will have a basic ingredient for several recipes.

That Fat-Soaked Gravy

Obviously gravy is off limits, particularly gravies made with fat and flour. But there *is* an alternative. To replace the fat and flour needed to thicken most gravies, Heather suggests using a fat-free veal stock. The stock thickens by itself when it is reduced by simmering because it contains natural gelatin. Try Wild Mushroom Sauce (p. 161) and Raspberry Sauce (p. 162) next time you need a gravy. And many of the stewed meats, and even the fish dishes, in this book are made from a rich, fat-free Low-Sodium Chicken Stock (p. 88).

A Little Can Go a Long Way

Take heart. Our "no-no" list is not as long as you might think. Some foods that seem to be off limits because of their fat content can provide a lot of flavor—and little fat—if used in *very* small quantities. A pinch (or half teaspoon) of coconut flakes only has .4 grams of fat and a teaspoon of roasted pecans has approximately 1 gram. Recipes like Baked Spiced Bananas (p. 215) only use a pinch of coconut, for instance, and Sole and Pecan Rolls (p. 185) uses a very small amount of pecans. Celery Cabbage with Ginger and Red Grapes (p. 142) uses a dusting of ground peanuts, which provides a nice flavor and a natural sweetness. Just a half teaspoon of freshly grated Parmesan cheese provides a great deal of flavor to soups, sauces, or pasta dishes, with only 29 grams of sodium and .6 grams of fat. A very small amount can go a long way, as the old saying goes. Be careful, though: If you are inclined to overindulge in these condiments, it may be better to expel them from your kitchen forever.

2. Eat More High Fiber Foods

Breakfast is the time of the day to concentrate on increasing your fiber intake. Granolas are packed with fiber, and Heather advises that cooks be creative with recipes like Granola with Fruits (p. 97) and add their own mixture of bran (or wheat germ), oats, barley, or any other grain. She also uses whole wheat flour and bran in Maple Breakfast Scones (p. 100) and whole wheat flour in Sweet Potato and Date Coffee Cake (p. 102).

To carry this high-fiber diet throughout the day, Heather has included several recipes for legumes, like Curried Black Beans (p. 109), Black Beans with Jalapeño and Orange (p. 108), and Spicy White Lima Beans (p. 107), all of which are high in fiber and can be served as main courses or side dishes. And it's no coincidence that many desserts in Part Two use fresh fruits, like Baked Spiced Bananas (p. 215), since fresh fruits are high in fiber and vitamins.

3. Consume Less Salt

People who suffer from kidney disease often have to go without salt altogether—or to accept one of the lackluster substitutes. They wonder, "How can I eat an egg without salt?" You may also be wondering, "How can I lower my salt intake without destroying the taste of my food? Where will I get the flavor?"

Chefs know that condiments prepared from herbs and other naturally low-sodium flavoring agents, such as chicken stock and garlic, can easily replace salt. If these flavoring agents are new to you, the recipes in this book will give you a glimpse of how tasty recipes prepared with these ingredients can be. For instance, Tomato Rosemary Sauce (p. 160) is a basic tomato sauce without added salt or sugar. The carrot adds some carotene (a form of vitamin A) and reduces the need for salt and sugar. Another option is to flavor your food with homemade stocks.

Flavor with Homemade Stocks

Homemade stocks—whether chicken, fish, beef, veal, or vegetable (see Vegetable Stock, p. 90)—provide an amazing source of flavor. If you refrigerate the stock, allow the fat to rise to the top and harden, and then skim it off before you use the stock, you will avoid the harmful effects of the fat content.

Stocks do take time to cook (from two to eight hours), but the actual time that you must stand by the stove is minimal, since their preparation just takes a few steps. You can prepare stocks while you cook something else or as you are sweeping and dusting the downstairs or even as you watch television. A timer can remind you to check the stock every once in a while. If you make a large stock—and use it to flavor many different recipes—the actual preparation time per dish isn't much at all. Stocks can be frozen for future use in plastic containers of cup, pint, or quart sizes, so you can make them once a month.

If you opt for the "quick-and-easy" method of purchasing commercial stocks, avoid canned stocks, which usually do not have good flavor. While a canned low-sodium broth is nutritional, you will probably notice that the added flavor does not compensate for the lack of salt. If you must use canned stocks, plan on amplifying the flavor with additional vegetables and herbs (see Fortified Canned Chicken Stock, p. 89). You do, however, have another alternative. Most gourmet markets sell fresh, homemade stocks. Be sure to read the labels to see that these stocks have no salt or additives.

Seasoning Vegetables

Nothing is tastier or more satisfying than corn-on-the-cob, picked just minutes before it's plunged into the pot, or fresh spring snap peas, right from the garden. Starting from this naturally flavorful foundation, extra taste can be added with fresh or dried herbs, spices, and fruits. In Bok Choy with Ginger and Apples (p. 141), for instance, the kumquats and apples complement the ginger to give the bok choy added taste. The fruit also adds a hint of sweetness and a refreshing texture. This touch of sweetness often satisfies that salt craving.

Flavoring agents such as these may seem to add too much cooking time if they are unfamiliar to you, but they can be just as fast and often more interesting than their salty counterparts. Sodium-rich sauces often mask the subtle flavors of fresh produce, rather than enhancing them. The recipes in Part Two of this book depend upon these sources of flavor, which are lower in sodium and fat.

Often vegetables that have been picked minutes or even hours before serving and are steamed need little more than a squeeze of lemon and a shake of black pepper to make them taste great. Some vegetable recipes in this book require little more effort than that flick of the pepper can, such as Brussels Sprouts with Caraway (page 153). In general our vegetable recipes only require the assembly of a few chopped ingredients with some herbs and spices, so they are relatively quick.

Another way to enrich the flavor of many vegetables is to brush an all-purpose dressing or sauce, such as Herbed Garlic Dressing (p. 169) or Lemon Tarragon Dressing (p. 170), over steaming hot vegetables. Many of the vinaigrette dressings, such as Shallot Vinaigrette (p. 174) and Papaya Coconut Dressing (p. 172), can also turn leftover chilled vegetables into a lovely salad like Broccoli Vinaigrette (p. 115). You might want to keep a variety of raw or steamed-and-chilled vegetables on hand so you can quickly prepare a vegetable for lunch or dinner—and don't forget to serve these vegetables as an easy, nutritious snack with a dip.

4. Eat Foods With Fewer Additives and Artificial-sounding Ingredients

In order to avoid preservatives and additives, you are going to have to prepare dishes from scratch. "The purest, most unique, and healthiest flavor comes from fresh unprocessed foods," Heather recommends. At the same time she realizes the tight schedules of most working people, like herself, and homemakers. Her solution? Prepare double recipes of basic sauces and stocks and dishes ahead of time that can be used for more than one recipe, such as Curried Black Beans (p. 109), which can be a main course or a hot dip or a side dish. Or make a double batch of Herbed Garlic Dressing (p. 169), which freezes well. You freeze half of it for a few weeks, then let the frozen half thaw in the refrigerator overnight before you use it. Be sure to blend the ingredients well before serving. The two brown sauces, Wild Mushroom Sauce and Raspberry Sauce, will also freeze well, as will any sauce that is made from a stock and is free of added dairy products.

The good news here is that fresh produce doesn't need additives. You can find wonderful flavor and more nutrients from fresh produce than from the canned, dried, or frozen varieties. To keep the best flavor, fresh produce should go directly from the garden into the pan. That natural flavor—and those nutrients—disappear all too quickly once the produce is stored, frozen, canned, or packaged.

That's why manufacturers seek to enhance vegetables with monosodium glutamate. Packaged foods also contain sodium-rich additives like sodium phosphate, sodium bisulfite, and sodium saccharin.

How to Select Fresh Produce

Vegetables are freshest when they are ripe, yet still firm, with taut skins. For example, green beans should not show any signs of dehydration (that telltale shriveled look), and tomatoes should have tight skins. If the outer edges of the stem of any vegetable have begun to shrivel and dry, the vegetable has been stored for too many days. The flowers on broccoli should be closed rather than in a yellow bloom.

In general, cabbages should be tight at the base. Look at the outer leaves. If any are missing from either cabbage or lettuce, the grocer has removed them to keep the deterioration from being noticeable. All herbs should be free from mold and dehydration and ideally as crisp as your lettuce.

Fruit that is less than fresh is even more easily detected. Apples, in particular, become overripe and soft and often begin to bruise, mold, or take on a fermented smell. Any sign of mold is a warning that the fruit or vegetable has lost both natural nutrients and flavor.

Herbs as Natural Additives

Fresh herbs, rather than dried, offer more complex flavors and aromas to your cooking, which will also make the use of additives and artificial ingredients unnecessary. Fresh basil loses much of its anise quality when it is dried and rosemary loses most of its scent. Even if you carefully tend your herb garden in the summer, or have access to fresh herbs at your local grocery market, you will probably have to use dried herbs during some winter months. Dried herbs are good enough and often cheaper for long-stewed dishes, and are an adequate substitute when fresh herbs are not available.

With these four major guidelines as benchmarks, Heather also considered two factors that have the double benefit of reducing your susceptibility to two of these diseases as she created the three-in-one recipes.

DOUBLE BENEFITS

As you were reading Chapters 2, 3, and 4, you may have noticed that one factor occurred in more than one chapter as a significant disease deterrent. You can reduce your susceptibility to heart attack and cancer if you *eat more foods that lower blood cholesterol.*

Eat More Foods That Lower Blood Cholesterol

Doctors tell heart patients to consider foods and ingredients that will reduce their cholesterol level. Two ingredients are particularly effective: Omega-3 fatty acids (found in fish) and olive oil.

Omega-3

Heather has included ten fish recipes in Part Two, particularly grouper (see p. 183 for Grouper with Sweet Peppers and Potatoes) and salmon (see pp. 177 and 178 for Poached Salmon Fillet and Salmon with Potato Crust), which are high in Omega-3 fatty acids. Be sure to choose fresh fish. Then add sauces and relishes, like Papaya and Citrus Relish (p. 165) or Black Bean and Banana Relish (p. 166).

Olive Oil

All of the vinaigrettes and many of the vegetable recipes suggest cooking with extra virgin olive oil. (Heather recommends extra virgin olive oil because this oil comes from the first pressing and, therefore, has a purer flavor than oil taken from later pressings.) If you do not like the robust flavor of olive oil, try "lite" olive oils, which are available at many markets. You can use olive oil for sautéing because the flavor will be lightened in the cooking.

The final factors that Heather considered as she developed the three-in-one recipes in Part Two were the important factors in reducing your susceptibility to cancer, which should not be overlooked.

MAJOR FACTORS FOR REDUCING YOUR SUSCEPTIBILITY TO CANCER

The American Cancer Society often advertises, "A defense against cancer can be cooked up in your kitchen." They particularly recommend eating:

1. Cruciferous vegetables such as cabbage, broccoli, cauliflower, brussels sprouts, kale, collard greens, turnips, rutabagas

2. Foods high in:

• beta-carotene, a form of vitamin A (dark green leafy vegetables, carrots, spinach, broccoli, sweet potatoes, peaches, apricots, cantaloupes)

• vitamin C (broccoli, cauliflower, sweet peppers, oranges, papaya, mangos, melons)

1. Eat More Cruciferous Vegetables

Cabbage is a mainstay of cancer prevention and a deterrent to strokes, since it is high in carbohydrates. To increase your cabbage consumption—and still maintain both nutritional and psychological diversity—Heather suggests that you try different varieties of this vegetable: bok choy or Chinese cabbage, celery cabbage, red cabbage, savoy cabbage, or napa cabbage. Each of them is delightful in its own way. For instance, bok choy and napa cabbages are lighter in flavor than traditional green and red cabbage, and celery cabbage has a hint of the flavor that gives it its name.

And there are many varieties of dark green, leafy vegetables: spinach, kale, mustard greens, collard greens, beet greens, and even broccoli greens (the leaves most people throw away—save them, they're good for you). Any of these green leafy vegetables can be used with salad recipes in this book, such as Collard Green Salad (p. 119). Be sure to steam kale, mustard greens, collard greens, beet greens, and broccoli greens, because they are tougher than lettuce and spinach. (See Steaming Vegetables, p. 87, for the steaming times for these greens.) Steamed greens can be served hot or chilled with a number of vinaigrettes, such as Papaya Coconut Dressing (p. 172) or Shallot Vinaigrette (p. 174).

If you have a gourmet supermarket in your area, explore the variety of produce that is available there. Then ask your local grocers to carry some of these greens if at all possible (they may be more agreeable than you think, but only at specific times of the year). Many times the local farmer's roadside stand or farmers' market supplies the freshest greens so be sure to add these markets to your summertime grocery shopping trips.

2. Foods High in Beta-Carotene and Vitamin C

Mother Nature has created many vegetables that are high in beta-carotene and vitamin C: broccoli, red peppers, those dark green leafy cruciferous vegetables, and papaya. Other cruciferous vegetables are high in vitamin C and/or vitamin A: cauliflower, cabbage, and bok choy. Many fresh herbs are good for more than just flavor. For instance, chili powder, cayenne pepper, and parsley are higher in vitamin A than other spices.

The citrus fruits, bell peppers, and the exotic fruits (like papaya, mango, and kiwi fruit) are all very high in vitamin C and make great foundations for sauces to be used with main courses or desserts: Mango Sauce (p. 218) as an accompaniment to Raspberry Turnover (p. 210) or to fruit or frozen yogurt; and Papaya and Citrus Relish (p. 165) as a garnish for fish or as a dip. Other relishes, like Fresh Tomato Salsa, can also be used as dips or snacks.

Though a spoonful of papaya or red pepper in a relish may not provide a large amount of vitamin C, you can incorporate relishes like Papaya and Citrus Relish (p. 165) into your diet as a sauce for dinner or as a salsa for snacking to further your protection. Every little bit helps.

Many of the recipes in Part Two give you the three-in-one benefit and also incorporate some of these special guidelines, as does Sweet Potato and Date Coffee Cake (p. 102). The beta-carotene in the sweet potato helps to reduce your susceptibility to cancer, the fiber and the nutrients of the whole wheat flour protect you from all three diseases, and the treat is almost nonfat and very low in sodium, a further three-in-one benefit.

THE THREE-IN-ONE MEAL

Heather's major goal in creating these recipes was to choose recipes that could be combined in various ways to provide preventive measures for all three diseases in one meal. Sometimes, it is impossible for one dish, like a roast of pork tenderloin, to be truly "three-in-one." A pork tenderloin roast is lower in fat and cholesterol than many other cuts of meat, but what nutrients does that roast have to prevent cancer?

Recipes like a pork roast will have the "three-in-one" benefit when they are combined with another dish or two into an entire meal plan, and that choice can be yours. The pork roast can be accompanied by Roasted Red Pepper Relish (p. 163) and a vegetable like steamed spinach. Then the entire meal fulfills the three-in-one goal. The relish provides vitamin C, and the spinach is high in beta-carotene.

Another example of a three-in-one meal is baked fish with Papaya and Citrus Relish (p. 165) accompanied by a Winter Garden Vegetable Salad with brussels sprouts (p. 122). The cruciferous vegetable is cancer preventative, as is the vitamin C in both the relish and the kumquats in the salad.

As you grow more familiar with the benefits provided by different foods and ingredients, it will become second nature for you to satisfy all three goals on a daily basis. To start you on that journey, here is a suggested daily menu with extra breakfast and lunch menus.

Daily Menu

Maple Apple Oatmeal
Fruit Salad

Whole Wheat Pita Sandwich with Curried Chicken Salad
Carrot Soup
Collard Green Salad

Roasted Pork with Kale and Goat Cheese
Curried Butternut Squash
Boston Lettuce with Apricot and Sage Dressing
Baby Bliss Potatoes with Parsley
Crusty Italian Bread

Vanilla Pudding with Blueberry Sauce

	Fat	*Cholesterol*	*Sodium*	*Calories*
Per Serving	46.9	143.7	628.8	1665.2

■

Breakfast Menu

Sweet Potato and Date Coffee Cake
Fruit Salad with Nonfat Yogurt

■

Luncheon Menu

Broccoli Vinaigrette
White Pizza with Rosemary

Start with this daily menu, and then create your own. Heather has designed these recipes to be interchangeable. One newly learned recipe can be combined with several different recipes in this book, rather than with only one specific dish. For instance, if you have a favorite whitefish, which is a low-fat/low-sodium main course, you might serve it with a sauce like Dill Sauce (p. 158). Or Horseradish Sauce can be served with lower fat cuts of beef, like flank steak, or with baked potatoes. Or you might combine one of these recipes with a favorite of your own or a vegetable like Braised Sweet and Sour Cabbage (p. 143).

Obviously you can also use the three guidelines Heather used to create the three-in-one recipes as you select recipes from cookbooks and magazines and devise (or revise) some of your own recipes.

FOODS TO AVOID

As you do this, we suggest that you investigate the appendix to this book. Appendix 1 contains a list of the calorie, fat, and cholesterol content of more than 275 commonly used foods. We suggest that you skim through this list and draw a line through the foods that should be off limits. At the same time, circle foods that you should be eating more frequently. Then refer to this list every couple of months to see how you are doing and to refresh your memory.

Appendix 2 gives you two suggested low-cholesterol, low-saturated fat diets. Since reducing fat intake is one of the four factors common to reducing your susceptibility to all three diseases, you might want to consult these lists and the suggested general meal plans to see if your daily meals really are reducing your fat intake.

Appendix 3 gives you the sodium content of more than 180 foods. Again we suggest that you go through this list and draw a line through those foods that are "no-no's" and circle the foods that you should be cooking more frequently. Once you have that information, Appendix 4 gives you low-sodium diets of 500 milligrams, 2,000 milligrams, and 4,000 milligrams. Suggested meal plans accompany each of these diets.

THE NATURAL PROCESS OF THREE-IN-ONE

Three-in-one cooking can become a natural process if we can learn to enjoy meats and fish that are lowest in fat and cholesterol, and sauces low in fat and sodium, like a fruit sauce for fish, and a salad dressing made from fruit nectar. Even Mom's spaghetti can be made from fresh tomatoes or canned tomatoes that have no added sodium and Sun-dried Tomato Paste (p. 95), which has a more interesting flavor than canned tomato paste and is lower in acid, requiring less salt.

The recipes in Part Two will prove to you that you can still have both familiar flavors and exciting new varieties—and relative ease in preparation. Deprivation and boredom do not have to go hand-in-hand with healthful eating. Yes, you are going to eat more cabbage, oats, fish, and chicken. But you are also going to enjoy White Pizza with Rosemary, coffee milkshakes, and Special Hamburgers with Peppered Yam Fries! You can live better, longer, with the three-in-one diet.

Part Two

Three-in-One Recipes to Save Your Life

Steamed Vegetables

Steaming time varies depending on the type of vegetable and how it's cut. Use this as a guide, and develop your own timetable depending upon how you prefer to prepare your vegetables.

Always wash your vegetables thoroughly. For greens such as spinach or kale, soak them in two separate baths to remove any sand or lodged debris.

When cutting vegetables for steaming, attempt to create uniform sizes. If that isn't possible, keep the smallest pieces aside and add them to the pot last. For broccoli stems, either split them in half or quarters, or slice them in 1/4-inch pieces.

Use a conventional steaming rack or place a small colander inside a pan. Always use a pan with a tight fitting lid.

Heat 1/2 inch to 3/4 inch of water to boiling with the cover on. The water should just touch the underside of the steaming basket. For steaming times longer than 3 minutes, check the water level periodically and add more if necessary.

Add your vegetables, placing the stems in first or facing down whenever possible. These receive the steam first, which they need since they are tougher. Add the smallest pieces on top.

Steam dark green leafy vegetables (greens) until they are just wilted and tender. Steam tougher vegetables like beans, asparagus and broccoli until the toughest portion is tender to taste yet still firm.

To keep the steamed vegetables from cooking further, serve immediately or remove them to their serving dish and cover. Or, if you plan to serve them chilled, remove them to an ice bath or the refrigerator.

These are approximate steaming times:

spinach leaves	**2–3 minutes**
greens	**4–6 minutes**
broccoli	**5–7 minutes**
green beans, asparagus	**8–10 minutes**
carrots	**10–15 minutes**
acorn squash, cut in half	**15 minutes**
spaghetti squash, cut in half	**15 minutes**

Thickest Yogurt

This method of thickening nonfat yogurt produces a sour cream look-alike without the fat or additives of sour cream substitutes. If you add fruit or other flavorings, the method produces a rich creamy pudding or topping for desserts. This recipe can be made from a pint or quart of yogurt.

1 cup nonfat plain yogurt
medium sieve
cheesecloth

Line a large rustproof sieve or colander with a double thickness of cotton mesh cheesecloth. (If you don't have access to cheesecloth, sterile gauze or coffee filters will work.) Place the sieve over a bowl large enough to collect 1/2 cup of whey (or half as much whey as yogurt).

Place the yogurt in the sieve, cover, and let rest in the refrigerator for at least 6 hours. The liquid will drain out, creating a thickened yogurt one half the volume of the original.

MAKES 8 tablespoons (or 1/2 cup)

	Fat (g)	Cholesterol (g)	Sodium (mg)	Calories
Total Recipe	0	0	162	108
Per Portion	0	0	27	18

Low-Sodium Chicken Stock

Chicken stock is most often made from a collection of chicken bones. This is an easy way to make fresh chicken stock without saving the bones in the freezer. Removing the breast meat when done also offers low-fat, tender meat for sandwiches and salads. By making your own chicken stock, you avoid any added sodium or other additives of canned broth while you amplify the nutrients with vegetables. And as far as flavor goes, you cannot find the richness of homemade stock in a can. That richness reduces the need for added sodium.

3 to 3 1/2-pound frying chicken
4 cups onion, cut into 1-inch pieces
2 cups carrot, cut into 1-inch pieces
1 cup celery, cut into 1-inch pieces

4 quarts cold water
1 teaspoon dried leaf thyme
1 bay leaf

Remove all skin and visible fat from the chicken.

Bring all ingredients to a simmer in a large pan, making sure the ingredients are covered with water. Do not boil the stock or it will turn cloudy.

Cook at a simmer for 35 minutes and remove the breast meat for use in other recipes.

Cook the stock for 1¾ to 2 hours further.

Strain the stock; reserve the carrots for use in two salad dressings in this book (see Carrot and Tarragon Vinaigrette and Apricot Sage Dressing). Remove and discard bay leaf. Cool the stock in the refrigerator until the fat rises to top. Skim all fat and refrigerate.

Use the stock within several days or freeze it in well-sealed 1- to 2-cup containers.

MAKES 16 cups

	Fat (g)	Cholesterol (g)	Sodium (mg)	Calories
Total Recipe	24	0	304	736
Per Portion	1.5	0	76	46

Fortified Canned Chicken Stock

Making your own chicken broth or stock will improve the flavor and nutritional content of your recipes beyond belief. But if you must use canned broth, it needs fortification. Canned broth alone cannot provide the flavor and richness needed to create robust recipes without added salt. You will probably find that it is just as easy to make the stock from scratch. This recipe can easily be doubled. If you have any bare raw chicken bones, a few added to this recipe will intensify its flavor.

16 ounces low-sodium canned chicken broth
½ cup chopped onion, cut into ⅓-inch pieces
¼ cup diced carrot, cut into ⅓-inch pieces
2 tablespoons diced celery, cut into ⅓-inch pieces
¼ teaspoon dried leaf thyme
½ bay leaf

Combine the ingredients and cook for at least 1½ hours. Remove and discard the bay leaf. Strain the broth and chill. Remove hardened fat from top.

MAKES 4 (½ cup) servings

	Fat (g)	Cholesterol (g)	Sodium (mg)	Calories
Total Recipe	3	0	152	92
Per Portion	.75	0	38	23

Vegetable Stock

If you choose to omit meat from your diet or don't have any chicken and need a stock, use this rich vegetable stock instead. It is fat free and low in sodium and calories. Chances are, you'll need to double the recipe.

3 cups onion, cut into ½-inch pieces
2 cups carrot, cut into ½-inch pieces
1 cup celery, cut into ½-inch pieces
3 cloves of fresh garlic, peeled
½ teaspoon dried leaf thyme
1 bay leaf
12 black peppercorns
parsley stems
2 quarts water

Combine the ingredients and bring to a boil. The vegetables should be well covered with water. Reduce to a simmer and cook for 2 hours. The vegetables should become very soft.

Remove and discard bay leaf. Strain the stock and freeze in cup or pint containers the portions you won't use immediately.

MAKES 8 cups

	Fat (g)	Cholesterol (g)	Sodium (mg)	Calories
Total Recipe	0	0	608	232
Per Portion	0	0	76	29

Veal Stock

Veal stock is a low-fat foundation for the richest of brown sauces or gravies. The natural gelatin in the veal bones thickens the sauce without the need for added fat and flour. The naturally robust flavor of sauces made from the stock does not need additional salt. While the process seems lengthy, it requires little attention and most of it can take place while you do something else around the house. Set the timer to remind you to check on the stock. Ask your butcher to save and freeze the bones for you, especially the shank bones, which he can split.

> **4 pounds veal bones**
> **1–2 pounds lean veal trimmings**
> **3 medium onions**
> **2 large carrots**
> **1 rib of celery**
> **2 tablespoons no-salt tomato paste, store-bought, or Sun-Dried Tomato Paste (page 95)**
> **4 quarts water**
> **1 teaspoon dried leaf thyme**
> **1 bay leaf**
> **parsley stems**

Roast the bones in a metal roasting pan at 400° F for 1½–2 hours, turning periodically to brown the bones thoroughly. Place the onions, cut in half, facedown in the roasting pan for the last hour or so to caramelize them. Do not burn the bones or the onion.

Remove the bones and onion to a large stock pot and add the remaining ingredients. Tie the herbs in a piece of cheesecloth.

Meanwhile, pour all grease from the roasting pan and reheat the pan, adding the tomato paste and a small amount of water. Stir up the browned bone drippings as the pan heats and add this liquid to the stock pot.

Bring the stock to a simmer and cook at a low simmer for about 8 hours, skimming fat periodically. Add a little extra water if the level dips far below the bones. Do not boil or stir the stock; rather, loosen the ingredients with a long spoon to make sure they are not sticking to the bottom of the pan. Otherwise they will burn and make the stock bitter.

After 8 hours strain the stock, pressing the bones and vegetables to extract their juices. Be sure to remove and discard the herbs in cheesecloth. The stock should be rich in color.

Let the stock cool in the refrigerator and remove all the fat that rises to the surface. Freeze the stock in pint containers for future use.

MAKES 8 pints

	Fat (g)	Cholesterol (g)	Sodium (mg)	Calories
Total Recipe	24	0	2432	736
Per Cup	1.5	0	152	46

Basic Pie Crust

Most pie crusts contain a large proportion of shortening, which gives them their flaky nature. This one lacks much of the fat and has a crispy nature to it; the key is to work it as little as possible so that you don't make the dough tough. It works well with dessert pies and for stuffing dinner or appetizer pies.

1/4 cup unsalted margarine
2 cups unbleached, all-purpose flour
3/4 cup ice cold water

To prepare the crust you will need two dinner knives and a medium sized bowl, or a food processor fitted with a metal blade. Put the margarine and your bowl and knives, or processor bowl and blade, into the freezer for about 45 minutes. When the shortening has hardened, slice it into 1/4-inch cubes. Put the cubes back into the freezer if you aren't going to continue to the next step immediately.

If using the food processor, place the flour and cold margarine cubes inside and pulse them about 20 times. DO NOT run the machine continuously. If you are using a bowl, cut the cold margarine cubes into the flour with the knives, working as quickly as you can until the consistency is uniformly coarse. If you must stop, place the whole bowl in the freezer.

To the flour mixture, add 1/2 cup ice cold water a few tablespoons at a time and mix quickly with your fingers, or pulse the food processor 5 times. Add the remaining 1/4 cup water and mix quickly with your fingers, or use about 5 pulses in the food processor. The dough should start to form a ball; do not continue to mix the dough until it looks smooth, or it will become tough.

Empty the dough onto a lightly floured surface, and fold the dough over on itself, pressing the damp dough and shortening into any dry flour. The idea is to press it together, not to knead it. If it is sticky to the touch, dust with flour. When you have a mass that holds together, form it into a flat smooth circle about 1/2-inch thick.

Wrap the dough in plastic wrap or wax paper and refrigerate it for about 2 hours, or until cold and firm. It is now ready for rolling and will fit a 9-inch pie pan. The dough can be frozen if well wrapped.

Roll the dough into a circle on a floured surface. Fold the dough carefully in half and place it in the pie dish. Do not stretch the dough; rather lay it generously in the dish and press the corners into place. Trim or flute the edges and prick the bottom with a fork several times. Let the crust rest in the refrigerator for 15 minutes before baking.

If prebaking the dough, line it with waxed or pastry paper and weigh it down with dried beans or rice. For a prebaked shell, bake in a 400° F oven for 10–15 minutes, removing the paper and weights after 8 minutes; for a partially baked shell, bake for 8–10 minutes.

SERVES 6

	Fat (g)	Cholesterol (g)	Sodium (mg)	Calories
Total Recipe	20.4	0	2.8	632
Per Portion	3.4	0	.7	158

Pizza Dough

This pizza dough omits the salt and is higher in nutrition than most because of the addition of wheat germ. If you choose to add the salt, add 125 milligrams of sodium to each portion. Try Pizza Sauce (page 156) with part-skim mozzarella cheese and instead of salty toppings, use fresh herbs and thinly sliced onion. For a less traditional treat, try White Pizza with Rosemary (page 227), or Vegetarian Pizza (page 226).

1 package active dry yeast (1 tablespoon)
1 1/2 cups warm water (110° F–115° F)
1 teaspoon sugar
1/2 teaspoon salt (optional)
1 tablespoon olive oil
3 3/4 cups unbleached, all-purpose flour
4 tablespoons toasted wheat germ
vegetable oil spray

In a large bowl, dissolve the yeast and sugar thoroughly with 1/2 cup of the water and let rest until small bubbles appear, about 10 minutes. Or, if using a mixer with paddle and dough hook, this can be done in the mixer bowl.

Mix the flour with the wheat germ and salt, if desired.

Add the remaining water to the yeast mixture and begin to stir in the flour mixture, using the paddle on a mixer, or a wooden spoon. Add the flour one cup at a time and stop adding flour when the mixture pulls away from the sides of the bowl and is a workable mass.

Turn the dough onto a lightly floured surface, and knead for approximately 8–10 minutes, dusting with flour if the mass becomes sticky. If using a mixer, replace the paddle with the dough hook and knead for 3–5 minutes.

Stop kneading when the dough is soft and elastic, like the consistency of an ear lobe.

Form a smooth ball with the dough, place in a slightly oiled bowl, and turn the dough to coat all sides. Cover the bowl with a towel, put it in a warm place, and let rise for approximately 1 hour, or until doubled in size.

Empty the dough onto a lightly floured surface, punch the dough down, knead it a few times, and reform it into a ball.

The dough is ready for rolling and can be rolled as thin or thick as desired. The recipe makes twenty-four miniature pizzas or two medium pizzas. You can use the dough right away or freeze it well wrapped for last-minute snacks. If while rolling the dough it refuses to keep its shape, let it rest covered for a few minutes and start over.

Use your favorite toppings and bake the pizza on a pizza pan sprayed with vegetable oil spray, in a preheated 425° F oven for about fifteen minutes or until the crust and underside are golden brown and the toppings are cooked.

SERVES 8
2 slices per serving

	Fat (g)	Cholesterol (g)	Sodium (mg)	Calories
Total Recipe	24.8	0	13.6	1904
Per portion	3.1	0	1.7	238

Cilantro Pesto

This is a low-sodium way to flavor meats, pasta, sauces, and sandwiches. The extra virgin olive oil offers a great source of monounsaturated fat. The flavor is intense and goes a long way when mixed with hot rice and pasta, or spread over meat. (See Basmati Rice with Cilantro Pesto, page 110.)

1/4 cup roasted, unsalted pumpkin seeds
1/2 cup extra virgin olive oil
2 teaspoons minced garlic
2 cups loosely packed fresh cilantro leaves

Heat a medium, heavy, nonstick skillet over medium-high heat. When the pan is hot, add the pumpkin seeds and pan roast for about 5 minutes or until their aroma is released and they are just turning golden. Remove to a bowl.

In a food processor fitted with a metal blade, purée the oil and garlic until fine.

Add the cilantro and process until smooth.

Add the seeds and continue processing until mixture reaches a uniform consistency.

MAKES 8 tablespoons

	Fat (g)	Cholesterol (g)	Sodium (mg)	Calories
Total Recipe	92	0	367	1028
Per Portion	12	0	46	129

— Sun-Dried Tomato Paste —

This tomato paste can be stirred into hot pasta or used in Italian dishes. It is a low-sodium, low-calorie basic to use in place of the canned variety. For tomato mayonnaise, stir 1 tablespoon of the paste into 1/4 cup reduced-calorie mayonnaise and 1/4 cup Thickest Yogurt (page 88).

12 sun-dried tomato halves
1/2 cup water

In a small, nonaluminum saucepan, bring the tomatoes and water to a simmer and cook for about 15 minutes.

The tomatoes should be soft and the liquid reduced by about half. If the liquid evaporates too quickly, add a little more water.

In a food processor fitted with a metal blade, purée the tomatoes with the cooking liquid. Add water if the mixture is too thick to purée.

MAKES 6 tablespoons

	Fat (g)	Cholesterol (g)	Sodium (mg)	Calories
Total Recipe	1.2	0	39.6	96
Per Portion	.2	0	6.6	16

Berry Yogurt Drink

This drink is low in fat, sodium, and calories. The raspberries add a special taste and fiber, as well as vitamin C. Try it for breakfast. Depending on your sweet tooth, you can add more honey. And you can use any berry in place of raspberries. Try using a ripe banana and a few strawberries.

1 cup nonfat plain yogurt
1/2 cup raspberries, frozen or fresh
1/8 teaspoon ground cardamon
1/4 teaspoon ground cinnamon
pinch of fresh nutmeg
1 tablespoon honey, or to taste

Warm the honey slightly and blend it with the yogurt.
Blend all the ingredients in a blender or food processor.

SERVES 1
1 1/2 cups per serving

	Fat (g)	Cholesterol (g)	Sodium (mg)	Calories
Per Portion	.5	0	162	275

Banana Frothy

This is very low in fat and high in nutrition. Try it for a snack or for breakfast. It's fairly low in sodium and calories and has a nice crunch.

1 ripe banana
1/2 cup nonfat plain yogurt
1/2 cup skim milk
pinch of ground cinnamon or nutmeg
1 tablespoon toasted wheat germ

In the blender or in a food processor fitted with a metal blade, blend all of the ingredients except the wheat germ. For a very cold drink, peel and freeze the banana in a plastic bag. Allow it to partially thaw, enough to slice it into 5 or 6 pieces. Blend it with the remaining ingredients.

Pour into a tall glass and top with wheat germ.

SERVES 1

	Fat (g)	Cholesterol (g)	Sodium (mg)	Calories
Per Portion	2.3	2	145	258

Granola with Fruits

This granola is packed with fiber, but unlike most granolas, it lacks the fat and sugar. The recipe can be doubled and is very forgiving as far as substitutions go; try using unsalted dry-roasted sunflower seeds or almonds instead of pecans. Or create your own combination of dried fruits.

8 ounces mixed dried fruits (approximately 1/2 cup pitted prunes, 1/2 cup pears, 1/4 cup apples)
1 cup golden raisins
5 cups uncooked rolled oats
2 cups oat bran
3/4 cup chopped pecans (3 ounces)
1/2 cup honey

In a large bowl, mix the grains and nuts together.

In a small pan, warm the honey until it liquifies and drizzle it over the grains, tossing as you go.

Preheat the oven to 325° F. Divide the grain mixture into three parts and roast each part separately on a nonstick baking sheet. Spread the grain evenly onto a cookie sheet and roast for about 30 minutes, turning and stirring every 10 minutes. (Bring the grain from the edges to the center.)

Cool the grain thoroughly and toss with the dried fruit. You can freeze half if you don't eat it frequently. The recipe makes 14 cups.

SERVES 28
1/2 cup per serving

	Fat (g)	Cholesterol (g)	Sodium (mg)	Calories
Total Recipe	190.4	0	36.4	3724
Per Portion	6.8	0	1.3	133

—— Maple Apple Oatmeal ——

Oatmeal is low in sodium and calories. The addition of wheat germ increases the nutritional value of this version. The apples, maple syrup, and spice give the cereal a popular flavor.

vegetable oil spray
2 Granny Smith apples, peeled and sliced 1/4-inch thin
1 teaspoon vanilla extract
1 tablespoon pure maple syrup
1/16 teaspoon ground cinnamon (about 1 pinch)
2 tablespoons wheat germ
1 1/2 cups quick-cooking oats
3 cups water
1 cup skim milk

Spray a large non-stick sauté pan with vegetable oil spray and lay one layer of apples in the bottom of the pan. Cook them slowly on medium heat about 4 minutes on each side. Turn them when they are golden brown. They should be soft inside but not mushy.

Meanwhile boil the water and stir in the oatmeal. Bring to a simmer, add the vanilla, and cook for about 5 minutes, stirring occasionally.

Spoon the oatmeal into ceramic bowls and arrange the apples on top. Drizzle with the maple syrup and cinnamon and broil until the apples start to sizzle. Serve immediately with skim milk, 1/4 cup per serving.

SERVES 4

	Fat (g)	Cholesterol (g)	Sodium (mg)	Calories
Total Recipe	9.2	4	126	766
Per Portion	2.3	1	31.5	191.5

Wheat Germ Waffles

These waffles are lower in fat and sodium than most and are choles-terol free. They have the added benefit of wheat germ's nutrients. Serve them with fresh fruit and yogurt.

**1 tablespoon safflower, corn, or canola oil
1 cup nonfat plain yogurt
1/4 cup water
3/4 cup unbleached, all-purpose flour
1 teaspoon baking soda
3 tablespoons toasted wheat germ
2 egg whites, beaten until frothy
vegetable oil spray**

Preheat the waffle iron. Using large bowl and whisk, blend the yogurt, oil, and water together.

Mix the flour, baking soda, and wheat germ in as few strokes as possible.

With a large rubber spatula, fold in the frothy egg whites. Spray the waffle iron with vegetable oil spray. Proceed with preparing the waffles according to the directions with your waffle iron.

SERVES 4

	Fat (g)	Cholesterol (g)	Sodium (mg)	Calories
Total Recipe	18.92	0	1084	724
Per Portion	4.73	0	271	181

Maple Breakfast Scones

These scones are sweet and spicy and lack the fat of most scones. They are made with baking powder instead of soda, which helps to reduce their sodium content. Serve with Fruit with Spiced Cream (page 202) instead of butter or cream.

1½ cups unbleached, all-purpose flour
2 teaspoons baking powder
¼ teaspoon ground nutmeg
2 tablespoons unsalted margarine
¾ cup oat bran, or bran/oatmeal blend
½ cup skim milk
¼ cup light brown sugar
1 tablespoon pure maple syrup
1 egg
¼ cup raisins, optional
vegetable oil spray

Stir the flour, bran, baking powder, and nutmeg together. Cut the margarine into small cubes and cut into the flour mixture. You can rub it between your hands until it looks like coarse meal.

Beat the milk, brown sugar, maple syrup, and egg together.

Blend the two mixtures together with the raisins in as few strokes as possible. Add a little more flour if the dough becomes sticky. Knead it a few times, pressing it together. Too much handling will make a tough biscuit.

Drop spoonfuls onto a cookie sheet sprayed with vegetable oil spray and pat the dough down lightly with moistened fingers. Or roll the dough out to about ½ inch and cut out circles.

Preheat oven to 425° F and bake for about 10 minutes or until golden. The recipe makes 12 scones.

SERVES 6
2 scones per serving

	Fat (g)	Cholesterol (g)	Sodium (mg)	Calories
Total Recipe	24	276	1050	1212
Per Portion	4	46	175	202

Praline Coffee Cake

This coffee cake is truly as sinful tasting as those that are higher in fat. The bubbly, sweet pecans do the trick. To avoid cholesterol altogether, replace the whole egg with two egg whites.

1 package dry yeast (1 tablespoon)
1/4 cup warm water (110° F–115° F)
3/4 cup skim milk
2 tablespoons unsalted margarine
1/4 cup sugar
1/2 cup Thickest Yogurt (page 88)
1 teaspoon vanilla extract
1 cup light brown sugar
1/2 cup pecan pieces
1 egg, beaten (or 2 egg whites, beaten)
2–2 1/2 cups flour
vegetable oil spray

Dissolve the yeast thoroughly in the water and let it sit for about 10 minutes. It should start to bubble.

In a small pan, warm the milk and shortening until the shortening melts. Meanwhile, prepare the topping. Blend the brown sugar, yogurt, and vanilla until smooth; stir in the pecans.

Put the milk mixture in a bowl and stir in the sugar. Once the mixture has cooled to room temperature, add the yeast mixture. Beat in the beaten egg.

Stir in the flour and mix well. Add flour until you can lift the dough out of the bowl in one piece; it will be stickier than most bread doughs, but you may dust it with flour if it refuses to stay intact. Dip your fingers in water to keep them from sticking to the dough while you knead it. Knead for 10 minutes. If using a food processor fitted with the dough blade, pulse it about 20 times.

Spray a cake or tart pan with vegetable oil spray and spread the dough into it. Cover with the topping and let it rise about 1 hour. You can prepare the coffee cake up to this point the night before, and let it rise covered with film overnight in the refrigerator. If so, let it come to room temperature before baking.

Preheat oven to 350° F and bake for 30–35 minutes or until center is done.

SERVES 8

	Fat (g)	Cholesterol (g)	Sodium (mg)	Calories
Total Recipe	93	272	399	3120
Per Portion	11.6	34	49.8	390

Sweet Potato and Date Coffee Cake

This coffee cake tastes and smells a lot more sinful than it actually is. With the benefits of the beta-carotene from the sweet potato and the fiber and nutrients of stone-ground wheat, you can't go wrong. This coffee cake uses half of the dough provided by the recipe; use the other half to make dinner rolls.

2 tablespoons vinegar
2 cups skim milk
1 package active dry yeast (1 tablespoon)
pinch of sugar
4 tablespoons light brown sugar
5 1/2 cups whole wheat flour
2 teaspoons ground cinnamon
1 teaspoon nutmeg
1 cup cooked sweet potato
1/2 cup nonfat plain yogurt
1/2 cup brown sugar
1/2 cup chopped fresh dates
pinch of nutmeg
1 egg white, beaten

Stir the vinegar into the skim milk and let it sit for about 10 minutes; it will sour. Or you can use 2 cups plus 2 tablespoons of buttermilk instead.

Dissolve the yeast thoroughly with 1/2 cup of the soured milk and a pinch of sugar. Let the mixture rest until the yeast starts to bubble, about 10 minutes.

Combine the flour, brown sugar, 1 teaspoon of the cinnamon, and the nutmeg.

Purée the sweet potato with the milk: Either press the potato through a sieve into a large bowl and stir in the milk until well blended, or blend them in the food processor. There should be no large pieces of potato in the mixture.

Add the yeast to the milk mixture.

Blend two cups of the flour mixture into the milk mixture until smooth. Slowly add flour until the dough pulls away from the side of the bowl. If you're using a processor, pulse the dough. The dough may take more or less flour, depending on the moisture in the potato.

When the dough becomes a workable mass that no longer sticks to your hands, begin kneading. Knead for 10–15 minutes, dusting with flour when the dough becomes sticky to the fingers. Too much flour will make the dough tough, so only add flour if the dough is unmanageable. If using the food processor with the kneading blade, about 20–25 pulses should knead it sufficiently. Form the dough into a smooth ball.

Oil a large bowl, place the dough in it, and turn the dough to coat top and bottom with the oil. Cover with a towel or plastic wrap and let the dough rise for about an hour or until doubled in size.

Punch the dough down and knead for a few more minutes. Re-form the dough and let it rise in the bowl as above. To do this step overnight, place the covered bowl in the refrigerator.

This next step can also be prepared ahead and chilled overnight. Blend the yogurt and 1/2 cup brown sugar until well blended. Add the dates, the remaining teaspoon of cinnamon, and a pinch of nutmeg.

When you're ready to prepare the coffee cake, divide the dough in half. You can wrap half well and freeze it, make rolls out of it, or double the topping in the previous step and make a double batch of cake.

Roll out the dough into a circle about 3/4-inch thick. Place it on an oiled pizza pan or tart pan and pinch up the edges. Spread the topping in the center, reaching out to the edge. Brush the edges with egg white.

Preheat oven to 375° F and bake for 15 to 20 minutes. The center bottom should sound hollow when thumped.

SERVES 10

	Fat (g)	Cholesterol (g)	Sodium (mg)	Calories
Total Recipe	15	8	466	3328
Per Portion	1.5	.8	46.6	332.8

Risotto with Asparagus

Risotto is a rich and creamy "comfort food." Whereas it can be high in sodium and cheese, this one is satisfying and flavorful without the fat and calories. You must use arborio rice, which is hard and can endure the cooking and stirring. Your final product should have a tender and firm rice kernel, swimming in a creamy base. The rice should not explode or turn mushy. The secret is to cook the rice at a low-to-medium simmer, stirring frequently to release the creamy starch.

> 1 tablespoon extra virgin olive oil
> 1/2 cup onion, minced (about 1/2 medium onion)
> 1 cup arborio rice
> 1/2 cup Ariél brand dealcoholized premium dry white wine
> 1/4 teaspoon freshly ground black or white pepper
> 3 cups homemade Low-Sodium Chicken Stock (page 88)
> 1/2 pound asparagus, trimmed and cut in 1/2-inch pieces
> 3 tablespoons freshly grated Parmesan cheese

Heat the olive oil in a heavy, nonstick saucepan to medium-high heat and sauté the onion for about 2 minutes, until it starts to turn clear. Stir in the rice and coat it with the oil.

Add the wine and pepper and reduce the wine by half its volume.

Add 1 cup of the chicken stock and the asparagus and stir up from the bottom. Cook at a low-to-medium simmer, stirring every 30 seconds or so.

When the rice starts to show itself as the stock cooks away, stir in 1/4 cup of stock. Keep stirring the rice and adding 1/4 to 1/2 cup of stock when necessary, until finished.

The rice is finished when it is tender and firm and somewhat creamy. It should not be dry or sticky.

Fold the Parmesan cheese into the rice just before serving, reserving a small portion for the top of each serving.

SERVES 6

	Fat (g)	Cholesterol (g)	Sodium (mg)	Calories
Total Recipe	24.6	16.5	639	1066.8
Per Portion	4.1	2.75	106.5	177.8

Barley and Kale

Instead of simply a grain side dish, this recipe offers the flavor and nutrients of green leafy kale and carrots, while the barley helps reduce cholesterol. These flavors are smooth and soothing. You can serve it as a side dish or double up for a main course meal.

1 teaspoon extra virgin olive oil
1 shallot, chopped (a scant 1/4 cup)
1/2 cup Ariél brand dealcoholized premium dry white wine
2 cloves fresh garlic, chopped
1/2 cup finely diced carrot
1 cup dried pearl barley
4 cups homemade Low-Sodium Chicken Stock (page 88)
1/2 teaspoon ground coriander
1/2 bay leaf
1/2 teaspoon thyme leaves
1/2 teaspoon red pepper flakes
1/4 pound fresh kale, trimmed of stems and chopped
1 tablespoon red wine vinegar

In a medium, heavy, nonstick saucepan, heat the olive oil over medium-high heat. Add the shallots and sauté until they start to turn clear; do not let them brown.

Add the wine and let it reduce until nearly gone.

Add the garlic, carrots, and barley and stir to coat with the olive oil.

Add the chicken stock, herbs, and spices and bring to a low simmer. Cook for about 20 minutes, stirring occasionally, until the barley is tender but still firm.

Meanwhile, clean the kale, remove the stems, and slice it in 1/4-inch wide strips. Once the barley is tender but still firm, add the kale.

Cook about 3 minutes more or until the barley is soft but not mushy and the kale is dark green and tender. Remove and discard the bay leaf.

Stir in the red wine vinegar just before serving.

SERVES 9
1/2 cup per serving

	Fat (g)	Cholesterol (g)	Sodium (mg)	Calories
Total Recipe	13.1	0	400.5	1116.9
Per Portion	1.5	0	44.5	124.1

Curried Yellow Lentils

Lentils are naturally low in fat, calories, and sodium and high in fiber. This lentil dish is spicy and robust. Serve it with any mild raita, over basmati rice, or as a starch side dish. It is also delicious served as a stew with whole wheat pita bread. These lentils are available at Indian stores. If you can't find them, substitute the common lentil found in your supermarket.

1/2 cup Indian yellow lentils (mungdal)
1 1/2 cups water
1 teaspoon ground turmeric
1/2 teaspoon ground coriander
1/2 teaspoon ground cumin
1/4 teaspoon red pepper flakes
1/16 teaspoon ground cloves (about 1 large pinch)
1/16 teaspoon ground cinnamon (about 1 large pinch)
1/8 teaspoon cayenne, optional
1/2 teaspoon roasted cumin seeds
1 tablespoon fresh lemon juice

Wash the lentils in a small saucepan by filling the pan with cold water and pouring off the water, leaving the lentils behind. Repeat the process 4 or 5 times, or until the water is no longer cloudy.

In a medium saucepan, heat the water, lentils, and turmeric to a simmer.

Stir in the coriander, cumin, and red pepper flakes.

Cook at a very low simmer uncovered for about 30 minutes, stirring occasionally. The lentils should be soft but not mushy and have a soupy consistency.

Stir in the cloves and cinnamon and add the cayenne to taste.

Meanwhile heat a small, heavy, nonstick skillet over high heat. Spray with vegetable oil and reduce heat to medium high. Add the cumin seeds and pan-roast them. Stir occasionally to keep the seeds moving, until their aroma is released and they are just turning brown.

Stir the cumin seeds and the lemon juice into the lentils just before serving.

SERVES 4
1/2 cup per serving

	Fat (g)	Cholesterol (g)	Sodium (mg)	Calories
Total Recipe	.7	0	472.5	244.8
Per Portion	.2	0	118.1	61.2

— Spicy White Lima Beans —

These beans make a decadent stew with robust Tuscan flavors of rosemary, garlic, and red pepper. Lima beans are naturally low in sodium. If you choose to add the salt, add 143 milligrams of sodium per serving. These beans can be served as a stew or thick soup; or serve smaller portions as a side dish.

**1 pound small dried white lima beans
1 medium onion, chopped
1 tablespoon fresh chopped garlic
1 tablespoon olive oil
1 cup Ariél brand dealcoholized premium dry white wine
3 cups homemade Low-Sodium Chicken Stock (page 88)
1 bay leaf
3 teaspoons dried rosemary
1 teaspoon red pepper flakes
1/2 teaspoon salt, optional
1/4 teaspoon cayenne pepper
8 sun dried tomatoes, soaked in warm water until soft, and
     diced into 1/4-inch pieces**

Soak lima beans in 3 cups of water for 3 hours. Discard the soaking water.

In a large, heavy, nonstick stew pot, heat the olive oil until it is hot. Add the onion and garlic and sauté until the edges are softened.

Add white wine to the onions and simmer uncovered until the wine is reduced by half.

Add low sodium chicken stock, bay leaf, rosemary, red pepper flakes, cayenne pepper, and beans to the simmering onions. Cook at a low simmer for 1½ hours, stirring occasionally to keep the stew from sticking.

Add the tomato, stir the beans and cook for 1 hour more, or until the beans are tender. The stew should be soupy like a thick stew, rather than dry. If too much liquid has evaporated in the cooking process, add a little water. Remove and discard the bay leaf before serving.

SERVES 8
1 cup per serving

	Fat (g)	Cholesterol (g)	Sodium (mg)	Calories
Total Recipe	20	0	2050.4	1612
Per Portion	2.5	0	256.3	201.5

Black Beans with Orange and Jalapeño

Most black bean preparations use smoked meats and salt, while this recipe gets its flavor from subtle orange and jalapeño. Serve these beans as a main course with Basmati Rice with Cilantro (page 110). They are also delicious tossed with Shallot Vinaigrette (page 174) and served as a salad with lettuce and tomato.

vegetable oil spray
3/4 cup onion, chopped fine (about 1/2 large onion)
1 1/2 teaspoons minced fresh garlic
1 cup black beans, rinsed
1/2 teaspoon ground cumin
1/2 teaspoon ground coriander
1/4 teaspoon ground cayenne pepper
2 1/2 teaspoons jalapeño pepper, deseeded and chopped
(about 1 pepper)
1 bay leaf
1 teaspoon orange zest, all white pulp removed, chopped
fine
1/2 teaspoon freshly grated ginger root
2 cups Low-Sodium Chicken Stock (page 88)
2 cups water
2 tablespoons fresh cilantro, chopped, or 2 tablespoons
fresh chopped parsley and 1 teaspoon dried cilantro
(leaf coriander)

Heat a heavy soup pot sprayed with vegetable oil spray over medium-high heat. Sauté the onion and garlic for about 2 minutes. Do not brown them.

In preparing the orange zest, use a zester or remove the peel from the orange with a very sharp knife. Cut away all white pulp from the underside, or the stew will be bitter. To prepare the minced jalapeño pepper, wash the pepper, remove the stem, and slice lengthwise. Under cold running water, remove the seeds with a paring knife or your fingers.

After mincing the pepper, immediately wash your hands with soap and warm water.

Add the black beans and remaining ingredients, except the fresh cilantro, and bring to a simmer. Simmer uncovered for 1¼–1½ hours over low-to-medium heat, stirring occasionally. The beans should cook slowly to keep the liquid from evaporating too fast.

The beans are done when they are tender but still intact and round, swimming in a soupy sauce. If the liquid evaporates too quickly, add a little water.

Stir in fresh cilantro to taste just before serving.

SERVES 6

¾ cup per serving

	Fat (g)	Cholesterol (g)	Sodium (mg)	Calories
Total Recipe	6	0	211.8	919.2
Per Portion	1	0	35.3	153.2

—— Curried Black Beans ——

As a main course or side dish, this can be served with any raita or yogurt-based cold sauce, like Yogurt with Mint, Chili, and Onion (page 157). Or, serve with Carrot Salad with Raita (page 120). Or turn the Indian flavors around and serve with Mexican accompaniments such as Fresh Tomato Salsa (page 168) and Thickest Yogurt (page 88) instead of sour cream.

vegetable oil spray
¾ cup chopped onion
1½ teaspoons minced fresh garlic
1 cup black beans, rinsed
½ teaspoon ground cumin
1 teaspoon ground coriander
¼ teaspoon ground cayenne pepper
1 teaspoon ground ginger
2 cups Low-Sodium Chicken Stock (see page 88)
2 cups water
⅛ teaspoon ground cloves (about 2 pinches)
⅛ teaspoon ground cinnamon (about 2 pinches)
2 tablespoons fresh chopped cilantro, or 2 tablespoons
**   chopped fresh parsley and 1 teaspoon dried cilantro**
**   (leaf coriander)**

Heat a heavy soup pot over medium-high heat and spray with vegetable oil spray. Sauté the onion and garlic for about 2 minutes. Do not brown them.

Add the black beans and remaining ingredients, except the fresh cilantro, cloves, and cinnamon and bring to a simmer.

Simmer uncovered over low–medium heat for 1¼–1½ hours, stirring occasionally. The beans should cook slowly to keep the liquid from evaporating too quickly.

The beans are done when they are tender but still somewhat intact and round, swimming in a soupy sauce. If the liquid evaporates too quickly, add a little water.

Stir in the ground cloves and cinnamon. Just before serving, stir in the fresh cilantro.

SERVES 6

¾ cup per serving

	Fat (g)	Cholesterol (g)	Sodium (mg)	Calories
Total Recipe	6	0	206.4	905.4
Per Portion	1	0	34.4	150.9

Basmati Rice with Cilantro Pesto

Basmati rice is so fragrant that it makes a very pleasing side dish without any sauce, salt, or herbs; so a dab of Cilantro Pesto is all that is needed. It works very well with curried dishes and yogurt-based sauces. Basmati rice is available in Indian or Asian stores or in the gourmet market. The American grown version, called Texmati rice, is also available.

1 cup Basmati rice
2½ cups water
1 tablespoon Cilantro Pesto (page 94)

Wash the rice first by placing it in its cooking pan. Run cold water over the rice and slosh it around. Pour off the water and repeat for 5 washings. The water should start to lose its cloudiness.

Add 2½ cups of water, bring to a boil, stir once, and reduce the heat to low. Cook the rice very slowly, covered tightly, for about 10 minutes at a low simmer.

It should be al dente and not gummy. A good test is to try to smear one grain on the counter with your finger. Remove the pan from the heat and let rest covered, steaming passively for about 10 minutes.

Stir in the Cilantro Pesto and fluff with a fork before serving.

SERVES 4

1/2 cup per serving

	Fat (g)	Cholesterol (g)	Sodium (mg)	Calories
Total Recipe	8	0	94.8	729.2
Per Portion	2	0	23.7	182.3

– Basmati Rice with Roasted – Cumin Seed and Raisins

This version of Basmati rice is slightly sweet and aromatic. The preparation is low in sodium, fat, and calories and needs no other sauce. Serve it with curried dishes. Basmati rice is available in Indian and Asian stores and in the gourmet market.

1 cup Basmati rice
2¹/₂ cups water
1 teaspoon cumin seed
¹/₄ cup yellow raisins
vegetable oil spray

Wash the rice first by placing it in its cooking pan. Run cold water over the rice and slosh it around. Pour off the water, and repeat for 5 washings. The water should start to lose its cloudiness.

Add the water, bring to a boil, stir once and reduce the heat. Cook the rice covered tightly for about 10 minutes at a low simmer.

It should be al dente. A good test is to try to smear one grain on the counter with your finger. Remove it from the heat and let rest covered, steaming passively for about 10 minutes.

Meanwhile, spray a small skillet pan with vegetable oil spray and roast the cumin seed over medium-high heat for about 3 minutes, or until the seeds emit their aroma and turn slightly brown. Watch them carefully, stirring, because they will burn easily. When they are finished, remove to a small bowl to stop the cooking process.

Fold the raisins and cumin seeds into the resting rice and fluff with a fork before serving.

SERVES 4

1/2 cup per serving

	Fat (g)	Cholesterol (g)	Sodium (mg)	Calories
Total Recipe	1.2	0	12	625.2
Per Portion	.3	0	3	156.3

Fusilli with Two Cheeses

Fusilli is a corkscrew-shaped pasta, and the curls hold cheese nicely. Although this is a pasta and cheese dish, it is low in fat, sodium, and calories. A small amount of part-skim mozzarella and the aroma of Romano cheese go a long way. Serve this as a side dish.

1 tablespoon extra virgin olive oil
1 medium onion, cut into 1/4-inch pieces
1 tablespoon chopped fresh garlic
1/4 cup Ariél brand dealcoholized dry red wine
18 ounces low-sodium Italian tomatoes with juices, chopped
2 teaspoons chopped fresh oregano (or 1/4 teaspoon dried oregano)
1/2 pound fusilli
6 ounces part-skim mozzarella cheese, grated
3 tablespoons fresh grated Romano cheese or Parmesan cheese
vegetable oil spray

Preheat the oven to 350° F. Heat the oil over medium-high heat in a heavy saucepan. Sauté the onion and garlic for about 3 minutes. Do not brown.

Add the red wine and simmer until it has thickened to a syrup.

Add the tomato and juices and cook rapidly for about 20–25 minutes. The sauce should still be chunky and loose, neither watery nor pasty.

Stir in the oregano and set aside.

Meanwhile, cook the pasta until al dente, or tender but not soft. For fusilli, this is about 10 minutes. Drain the pasta.

Spray a baking dish with vegetable oil spray. Layer 1/3 of the pasta, 1/2 of the mozzarella, and 1/3 of the tomato sauce until finished, ending with tomato sauce. Cover the top with the Romano cheese.

Cook at 350° F until the cheese melts throughout.

SERVES 8

1/2 cup per serving

	Fat (g)	Cholesterol (g)	Sodium (mg)	Calories
Total Recipe	45.5	123.6	1728	1784
Per Portion	5.7	15.5	216	223

Fruit Salad

Readily available fruits can make a beautiful salad. The kiwi fruit and strawberries in this one are high in vitamin C. Keep a fresh fruit salad on hand for breakfast, lunch, dessert, or snacks.

2 cups quartered strawberries
1 cup seedless red grapes
1 Granny Smith apple, cored and diced
juice of 1 lemon
1 pear, cored and diced
2 kiwi fruit, peeled and sliced 1/4-inch thin
sugar as needed
6 small fresh mint sprigs

Wash all the fruit thoroughly and leave the skin on, except for the kiwi fruit.

Drizzle the lemon juice over the apple and pear to keep them from turning brown.

If the strawberries are tart, sprinkle with a little sugar.

Toss all the fruit together and serve garnished with fresh mint.

SERVES 6
1 cup per serving

	Fat (g)	Cholesterol (g)	Sodium (mg)	Calories
Total Recipe	4.2	0	18	508.8
Per Portion	.7	0	3	84.8

——— Broccoli Vinaigrette ———

Asparagus is traditionally served in this manner, though any steamed and chilled vegetable is delicious this way. It is a great way to serve cruciferous vegetables such as broccoli and cauliflower or those high in beta-carotene such as carrots and the dark green leafy vegetables. Also try Collard Green Salad (page 119).

¹/₂ pound fresh broccoli
2 tablespoons extra virgin olive oil
2 tablespoons balsamic vinegar
2 teaspoons minced shallots
¹/₂ teaspoon freshly ground black pepper
2 teaspoons sugar

Trim the broccoli, removing the toughest part of the stem. Cut the broccoli into long spears, with equal-sized stems.

Steam the broccoli, stem side closest to the water, for about 5 minutes or until it is tender but still firm.

When done, remove it from the pan to stop the cooking and refrigerate on the serving plate.

Whisk or process the olive oil in a slow stream into the vinegar and shallots so that it emulsifies. Add the pepper and sugar.

Pour the vinaigrette over the cooled vegetables and let them sit at room temperature for about an hour before serving.

SERVES 6

	Fat (g)	Cholesterol (g)	Sodium (mg)	Calories
Total Recipe	28.2	0	74.4	357.6
Per Portion	4.7	0	12.4	59.6

— Green Beans Vinaigrette —

This vinaigrette is rich in flavor while being lower in salt than most. The extra virgin olive oil is a good source of monounsaturated fat.

1/2 pound green beans
2 tablespoons balsamic vinegar
2 tablespoons extra virgin olive oil
1/2 teaspoon sugar
1/4 teaspoon coarsely ground black pepper
1/4 teaspoon minced fresh garlic
2 teaspoons grated fresh Parmesan cheese

Wash and trim the ends from the beans. Steam the beans for about 10 minutes or until tender yet firm. Chill immediately in the refrigerator.

In a small bowl, whisk the garlic, sugar, pepper, and vinegar together until blended. Slowly whisk in the olive oil.

Toss the chilled beans with the vinaigrette and the Parmesan cheese.

SERVES 3
3/4 cup per serving

	Fat (g)	Cholesterol (g)	Sodium (mg)	Calories
Total Recipe	28.4	0	101.2	341.2
Per Portion	7.2	0	25.3	85.3

Sweet Napa Salad

This is a sweet and sour cabbage salad and a great source of the nutrients from the Cruciferous family. It is relatively low in sodium and calories. The fat it does provide is from olive oil, which is high in monounsaturates.

1/2 cup extra virgin olive oil
1/4 cup garlic-flavored vinegar, or champagne vinegar
1 tablespoon honey
1 large head Napa cabbage
1/2 cup raisins
1 teaspoon celery seed
1/8 teaspoon freshly ground black pepper

Whisk or process the olive oil in a slow stream into the vinegar so that it emulsifies. Add the honey in the same fashion and set the sauce aside.

Remove the stem from the cabbage and cut the leaves into 3/4-inch slices; just slice through the whole cabbage, moving from end to end. Wash it and drain well.

Toss the raisins and cabbage with the dressing. When the cabbage is coated evenly, toss in the celery seed and pepper.

SERVES 10

	Fat (g)	Cholesterol (g)	Sodium (mg)	Calories
Total Recipe	82	0	117	1132
Per Portion	8.2	0	11.7	113.2

Spicy Slaw with Cilantro and Jalapeño

This is a variation on traditional slaw. It goes well with any Southwestern or Mexican meal, as a side dish or on a sandwich. It uses both cabbage and carrot, high in beta-carotene and the other nutrients of the Cruciferous family. The sweet red pepper is high in vitamin C.

2½ teaspoons jalapeño pepper, seeded and minced (about 1 medium pepper)
½ teaspoon minced fresh garlic
½ cup nonfat plain yogurt
2 tablespoons reduced-calorie mayonnaise
2 tablespoons chopped fresh cilantro
½ teaspoon black pepper
2 teaspoons sugar
1 tablespoon rice vinegar, or 2 teaspoons red wine vinegar

1 cup shredded or chopped cabbage (about ¼ medium cabbage)
1 cup shredded carrot (2–3 medium carrots)
¾ cup minced sweet red pepper (about 1 small pepper)

To prepare the jalapeño pepper, wash it, remove the stem, and slice lengthwise. Under cold running water, remove the seeds with a paring knife or your fingers and mince the pepper fine. Immediately wash your hands with soap and warm water.

In a food processor fitted with a metal blade, blend the first group of ingredients together until smooth. If you like your slaw sweet, add more sugar.

Toss the cabbage, carrots, and sweet red pepper with the sauce and let rest for about an hour before serving, so the flavors can blend.

SERVES 6

	Fat (g)	Cholesterol (g)	Sodium (mg)	Calories
Total Recipe	9	0	295.8	234
Per Portion	1.5	0	49.3	39

Caraway Slaw

This is a traditional version of slaw without the fat, sodium, and calories. Enjoy the preventative nutrients of the cabbage and the carrots' beta-carotene. Serve it as you would cole slaw or try Focaccia with Slaw and Swiss (page 236). If you use low-sodium Dijon mustard, reduce the sodium content by 58 milligrams per serving.

1/2 cup Thickest Yogurt (page 88)
2 tablespoons reduced-calorie mayonnaise
1/2 teaspoon celery seed
1/2 teaspoon caraway seed
1 tablespoon Dijon mustard
2 teaspoons sugar

1 cup shredded or chopped cabbage (about 1/4 medium cabbage)
1 cup shredded carrot (2–3 medium carrots)

In a food processor fitted with a metal blade, blend the first group of ingredients together until quite smooth.

In a medium bowl, toss the cabbage and carrot with the sauce and let it rest in the refrigerator for at least an hour so the flavors can blend.

SERVES 6

	Fat (g)	Cholesterol (g)	Sodium (mg)	Calories
Total Recipe	12	0	825	298.2
Per Portion	2	0	137.5	49.7

Collard Green Salad

Like other greens, collards are high in beta-carotene and fiber. The sweet red pepper adds vitamin C. Young collard greens are one of the sweetest greens, so hunt for the smallest leaves.

1/2 pound collard greens
1/2 sweet red pepper
4 tablespoons Shallot Vinaigrette (page 174)

Wash and remove the stems from the greens. Slice them in 1/3-inch strips and then again into 4-inch pieces. Soak them a second time.

Remove the seeds and white pulp from the red pepper and cut into 1/8-inch strips.

Steam the greens for about 5 minutes, or until they are tender but not soft. This will vary depending on the age of the leaves.

Remove from the pan and chill immediately.

Just before serving, toss the sweet red pepper with the collards and then with the vinaigrette.

SERVES 4

	Fat (g)	Cholesterol (g)	Sodium (mg)	Calories
Total Recipe	9.2	0	86.8	172
Per Portion	2.3	0	21.7	43

—— Carrot Salad with Raita ——

This is a spicy Indian sauce, but not too hot. The carrots offer all the benefits of beta-carotene and the sauce is a nonfat, low-sodium accompaniment. They are delicious with any other curried dishes.

1/2 pound thin carrots
1/2 cup nonfat plain yogurt
1/4 cup cucumber, peeled and very finely diced (about 1/4
    medium cucumber)
1 tablespoon fresh cilantro, chopped
1/2 teaspoon ground cumin

Wash and peel the carrots and cut them in half. For larger pieces, cut into quarters.

Steam the carrots for about 10–15 minutes, depending on their size. Chill for 1 hour in the refrigerator.

Combine the other ingredients in a small bowl and chill for at least 1 hour in the refrigerator.

Serve the raita spooned on top of the carrots.

SERVES 4
1/2 cup per serving

	Fat (g)	Cholesterol (g)	Sodium (mg)	Calories
Total Recipe	.6	0	158.4	158.4
Per Portion	.15	0	39.6	39.6

— Cucumber Salad with Dill —

Serve this as a salad or without the ice as an accompaniment to fish like Yellowtail Sole with Sesame Seeds and Black Pepper (page 185).

2 cups cucumber slices, peeled and sliced wafer-thin (about 1 medium cucumber)
3 tablespoons balsamic vinegar
1 tablespoon extra virgin olive oil
· **2 tablespoons fresh dill, chopped, or 1 teaspoon dry dill weed**
1/4 teaspoon freshly ground black pepper

With a whisk blend the vinegar, dill, and pepper. Slowly whisk in the olive oil until well blended. Pour the dressing over the sliced cucumbers in their serving bowl. Marinate the cucumbers for about 15 minutes in the refrigerator.

Top with fresh dill sprigs and a few small ice cubes or chips before serving.

SERVES 4

1/2 cup per serving

	Fat (g)	Cholesterol (g)	Sodium (mg)	Calories
Total Recipe	14	0	13.2	163.2
Per Portion	3.5	0	3.3	40.8

Winter Garden Vegetable Salad

This salad takes advantage of the brussels sprout, a member of the Cruciferous family. The kumquats offer vitamin C. This is a good place to serve kumquats over the winter months, but make sure they are sweet. The best way to determine their sweetness is to sample one; ask your produce grocer to rinse one for you to try.

1/2 pound brussels sprouts
8 kumquats
1 tablespoon dried currants
2 tablespoons raspberry vinegar
1 tablespoon minced shallots
2 teaspoons sugar
2 tablespoons plus 1 teaspoon extra virgin olive oil

Trim any brown leaves from the brussels sprouts and trim the ends. Make a shallow cross in the stem, which will allow it to cook thoroughly.

Put the brussels sprouts in a medium, heavy, nonstick saucepan with a tightly fitting lid. The sprouts should fit rather tightly in the bottom of the pan, without a steaming basket. Add 1/4 inch of water. Let the stems rest in the water and cover the pan tightly. Cook them for 4–5 minutes; the stems will cook while the leaves steam. They should be cooked and pliable, but not soft. Remove them from the heat, drain, and chill in the refrigerator.

Wash the kumquats, slice them thinly, and remove any seeds you might see.

Cut the brussels sprouts in half and toss with the kumquats and currants.

With a whisk blend the vinegar, shallots, and sugar. Slowly whisk in the olive oil until the vinaigrette is frothy and well blended.

Toss the salad with the vinaigrette and let it sit for 30 minutes before serving.

SERVES 4

2/3 cup per serving

	Fat (g)	Cholesterol (g)	Sodium (mg)	Calories
Total Recipe	32	0	32.4	479.6
Per Portion	8	0	8.1	119.9

Curried Chicken Salad

This chicken salad is moist and creamy without the fat. Finely diced carrot adds crunch and sweetness while supplying beta-carotene.

3/4 cup nonfat plain yogurt
1 tablespoon reduced-calorie mayonnaise
1/4 cup finely chopped red onion, cut into 1/8-inch cubes
(about 1/4 medium onion)
1/3 cup finely chopped carrot, cut into 1/8-inch cubes (about
1 medium carrot)
1/3 cup finely chopped celery, cut into 1/8-inch cubes (about
1 small stalk)
2 cups chicken breast meat, in small cubes (from 1 pound
raw chicken)
1 tablespoon curry powder
1/8 teaspoon cayenne pepper or to taste
1/4 cup loosely packed raisins

Combine the yogurt, mayonnaise, and spices. Mix all ingredients together.

Refrigerate and adjust the cayenne to taste.

Try serving this salad cold on fresh spinach leaves as a luncheon salad, or as a sandwich with tomato and sprouts in pita bread.

SERVES 4

	Fat (g)	Cholesterol (g)	Sodium (mg)	Calories
Total Recipe	23.2	232	436	772
Per Portion	5.8	58	109	193

Mexican Salad

This salad has much of the appeal of most Mexican foods without as much fat, calories, and sodium as are normally associated with this cuisine. Serve the salad with Southwestern Cornbread (page 222) and Fresh Tomato Salsa (page 168) or Hot Sauce (page 155).

1/2 cup onion, chopped fine (about 1/2 medium onion)
1 tablespoon fresh garlic, minced
1 teaspoon sunflower, corn, canola, or light olive oil
3/4 pound ground round of beef
1 tablespoon chili powder
1/4 teaspoon cayenne pepper
1 tablespoon jalapeño pepper, minced
2 tablespoons Barbecue Sauce (page 154)
3 cups shredded leaf lettuce
1 medium tomato, chopped
1/4 cup low-sodium cheddar cheese, grated
2 tablespoons Thickest Yogurt (page 88)

Heat a heavy, nonstick skillet over medium-high heat and sauté the onion and garlic for about 3 minutes.

Turn the heat up to high and add the ground round, pushing the onion and garlic aside. Add the spices and jalapeño and brown the meat.

Place the meat in a sieve and let the fat drain off. In a bowl, stir in the barbecue sauce and set aside.

Arrange the lettuce and tomato on 4 plates and distribute the meat over each plate. Sprinkle with cheese and serve with a spoonful of yogurt.

SERVES 4

	Fat (g)	Cholesterol (g)	Sodium (mg)	Calories
Total Recipe	55.8	213	547.2	993
Per Portion	9.3	35.5	91.2	165.5

Cucumber Dill Soup

This is a cold soup that is rich-tasting and refreshing. Serve it before your main course instead of a salad, or with a sandwich for lunch. If you choose to prepare this soup the day before, reduce the garlic to 1 teaspoon; it will intensify over time and you can always add more.

1 large cucumber, peeled
1½ teaspoons chopped fresh garlic
½ cup nonfat plain yogurt
½ cup Low-Sodium Chicken Stock (see page 88)
⅛ teaspoon white pepper
1 tablespoon chopped fresh dill (or 1 teaspoon dried dill)

Process the cucumber and garlic in a food processor until chopped fine.

Add the yogurt, chicken stock, and pepper and continue blending until smooth.

Stir in the dill and let rest in the refrigerator for at least 1 hour.

Serve cold, garnished with fresh dill sprigs.

SERVES 4

¾ cup per serving

	Fat (g)	Cholesterol (g)	Sodium (mg)	Calories
Total Recipe	.8	0	123.6	102
Per Portion	.2	0	30.9	25.5

— Southwestern Gazpacho —

This cold summer soup is extremely low in sodium, fat, and calories. It is refreshing and slightly spicy. Try it as a first course instead of a salad. Use the ripest tomatoes you can find; using fresh cilantro is well worth it.

1 cup chopped green pepper
3 cups chopped tomato
1 1/2 teaspoons fresh minced garlic
1 tablespoon lime juice
1 tablespoon rice vinegar
1/2 teaspoon grated fresh ginger root
6 ounces no-salt mixed vegetable juice
3 scallions, dark green portion removed, sliced very fine
1/4 teaspoon freshly ground black pepper
1 tablespoon chopped fresh cilantro, or 1 tablespoon
    chopped fresh parsley plus 1 teaspoon dried cilantro
    (leaf coriander)
pinch cayenne or to taste

In a food processor or blender, mince the green pepper. Add the tomato, garlic, lime juice, vinegar, and ginger root. Process until all ingredients are equal-sized or until nearly smooth.

Stir in the juice, scallions, peppers, and cilantro. Let rest at least 2 hours.

Serve cold with fresh cilantro leaves.

SERVES 4

	Fat (g)	Cholesterol (g)	Sodium (mg)	Calories
Total Recipe	1.2	0	78.16	151.2
Per Portion	.3	0	19.5	37.8

Dilled Spinach Soup

This is a light soup and a different way to get the nutrients of dark green vegetables. The soup is delicious served cold if you delete the rice and stir in 1/2 cup of nonfat plain yogurt.

1/2 cup chopped onion
vegetable oil spray
1/2 pound fresh spinach
1/4 cup Ariél brand dealcoholized premium dry white wine
1/4 teaspoon dried thyme
1/4 cup rice, cooked until it is mushy
3 cups Low Sodium Chicken Stock (p. 88)
1/2 teaspoon dried thyme
1/2 teaspoon ground nutmeg
1/4 teaspoon ground white pepper
1 tablespoon fresh lemon juice
1 1/2 teaspoons dried dill, or to taste
4 teaspoons nonfat plain yogurt

Spray a medium saucepan with vegetable oil spray and sauté the onions on medium heat until the edges turn clear, about 7 minutes. If they start to brown, reduce the heat.

Remove the woody stems of the spinach and soak it in cold water for 5 minutes. Drain and soak again to remove any sand. Drain the spinach.

Add the wine to the pan and let it reduce to a syrup.

Add the spinach, stock, herbs, spices, and rice and simmer about 10 minutes. Too much heat will turn the spinach brown.

Purée the spinach mixture in a blender or food processor. Make sure all the rice is liquefied.

Return to the heat and add the nutmeg, white pepper, lemon juice, and dill. Reheat slowly, but do not boil.

Serve with a small spoonful of yogurt.

SERVES 4
1 cup per serving

	Fat (g)	Cholesterol (g)	Sodium (mg)	Calories
Total Recipe	5.6	0	587.6	326
Per Portion	1.4	0	25.9	81.5

Carrot Soup

This soup is a tasty way to enjoy the beta-carotene of carrots. The carrots have a naturally sweet and comforting flavor when stewed with stock and a little wine. Starting a meal with such a satisfying soup makes it easy to follow with a light meal.

1/2 cup chopped onion
3 tablespoons chopped shallots or 1 teaspoon fresh chopped garlic
1 teaspoon unsalted margarine
1/4 cup Ariél brand dealcoholized premium dry white wine
1/4 cup finely chopped celery
41/2 cups Low-Sodium Chicken Stock (page 88)
1/2 teaspoon dried leaf thyme
1/2 bay leaf
2 cups carrots, peeled and sliced thinly

In a medium saucepan, heat the margarine over medium high heat and add the onion and shallots. Reduce to low heat and let them brown slowly, cooking for about 8 minutes, stirring frequently. Allow them to caramelize, making sure they don't burn.

Add the wine and celery, and allow the wine to reduce to a syrup.

Add the carrots, stock, and herbs and bring to a simmer.

Simmer until the carrots are soft, about 1 hour.

Remove and discard the bay leaf and purée the soup in a blender or food processor.

Garnish with fresh thyme or a sprinkling of freshly grated Parmesan cheese.

SERVES 6
1 cup per serving

	Fat (g)	Cholesterol (g)	Sodium (mg)	Calories
Total Recipe	9	0	444.6	412.2
Per Portion	1.5	0	74.1	68.7

Asparagus Soup

This is a rich but low-fat soup which relies upon a homemade stock. With such a rich-tasting first course, it is easy to follow with a lighter meal. You may want to serve the soup without the milk and with a dusting of Parmesan cheese; in place of the milk, 1/2 teaspoon of grated cheese will add approximately 20 milligrams of sodium and .2 grams of additional fat per serving.

vegetable oil spray
1/2 cup finely chopped onion, about 1/2 medium onion
1/4 cup finely chopped celery
1/2 bay leaf
1/2 teaspoon dried leaf thyme
1/2 cup Ariél brand dealcoholized premium dry white wine
3 cups Low-Sodium Chicken Stock (page 88)
3 cups asparagus, cut into 1/2-inch pieces, about 1/2 pound
1 cup milk, 2 percent or low-fat

Spray a medium saucepan with vegetable oil spray, heat over medium-high heat, and sauté the onion until the edges are clear. Stir in the celery and herbs.

Add the wine and reduce until it is a syrup.

Add the asparagus and stock and simmer gently until tender, about 15 minutes.

Remove and discard the bay leaf and purée the soup in a blender or food processor. Reheat and, if desired, stir in 1 cup of milk.

SERVES 4

	Fat (g)	Cholesterol (g)	Sodium (mg)	Calories
Total Recipe	10.8	18	388	478
Per Portion	2.7	4.5	97	119.5

Curried Yellow Split Pea Soup

This is a spicy, comforting soup. It's a great way to enjoy a hearty meal. Serve it as a soup or with Basmati rice as a stew. (Basmati rice is an aromatic rice, originally from Asia and now available from the U.S. too.) It is delicious with a small spoonful of plain nonfat yogurt on top.

1½ cups chopped onion
¾ cup finely diced carrot
⅓ cup finely diced celery
3 teaspoons fresh chopped garlic
1 pound yellow split peas
½ bay leaf
1 teaspoon ground cumin
1 teaspoon ground coriander
1 teaspoon curry powder
¼ teaspoon red pepper flakes
¼ teaspoon ground cloves
½ teaspoon ground cinnamon
9 cups Low-Sodium Chicken Stock (see page 88)

Combine all ingredients in a soup pot and bring to a boil.

Reduce the heat to a low simmer and cook about 1 hour. The peas should be soft but not mushy.

Stir in 2 pinches of ground cloves and remove and discard bay leaf before serving.

SERVES 12
1 cup per serving

	Fat (g)	Cholesterol (g)	Sodium (mg)	Calories
Total Recipe	18	0	684	1366.8
Per Portion	1.5	0	57	113.9

Chili

Most chili is loaded with sodium and fat. This one is lower in fat because it uses turkey breasts. Lots of spice and cilantro replace salt and give plenty of flavor. Serve it with finely chopped red onion and a spoonful of Thickest Yogurt (page 88) instead of sour cream. It also goes well with Southwestern Corn Bread (page 222).

> 1 pound turkey breast, cut into 1/4-inch strips
> 1 teaspoon safflower, corn, soybean, canola or light olive oil
> 3 cups chopped onion
> 1 1/4 cups diced green pepper
> 4 cups no-salt-added kidney beans (2 5 1/2-ounce cans), or homemade, or use regular canned kidney beans, rinsed under cold running water
> 3 cups drained no-salt tomatoes (3 14 1/2-ounce cans), reserve tomato juices
> 2–3 large cloves of fresh garlic, chopped
> 3 tablespoons chili powder
> 1/8 teaspoon red pepper flakes
> 1 tablespoon Cilantro Pesto (page 94)
> 2 teaspoons sugar

Brown the turkey in a large nonstick skillet in three separate batches. Make sure the pan is hot each time. Remove each batch to a stew pot. Drain off any fat if it accumulates.

Add 1/2 cup of water to the empty skillet and simmer to reduce by one-half, scraping up the browned meat juices. Remove the juices to the stew pot.

Let the pan dry and then add the oil. Once the pan is hot, sauté the onion, allowing it to brown before stirring.

Add the green pepper and cook for 2–3 minutes longer.

Add the onion and green pepper to the pot along with the kidney beans, tomato, garlic, chili powder, and pepper flakes. Add the reserved tomato juice as needed throughout cooking.

Cook for 1 1/2 hours or until the meat is tender.

Before serving, stir in the Cilantro Pesto and sugar.

SERVES 8

	Fat (g)	Cholesterol (g)	Sodium (mg)	Calories
Total Recipe	32.8	234.4	2239.2	2085.6
Per Portion	4.1	29.3	279.9	260.7

Lentil Stew

Lentils are a good source of fiber. They make a great side dish or main course meal. This recipe is very low in sodium, fat, and calories. For a cold lentil salad, simply toss partially drained lentils with Shallot Vinaigrette (page 174) and serve over tender lettuce with tomato or your favorite salad vegetables. Unfortunately, lentils are often either served bland or overspiced. It's well worth the few extra seconds and pondering to taste and adjust the seasonings at the end of cooking; aim for equal hints of pepper, thyme, basil, and cloves.

1 pound dry lentils
2 quarts water
2 cups chopped onion, cut into 1/4-inch pieces (about 2
   medium onions)
2 cups diced carrot, cut into 1/4-inch pieces (about 3 medium
   carrots)
1 cup diced celery, cut into 1/4-inch pieces (about 11/2 ribs
   celery)
1/2 bay leaf
1/8 teaspoon red pepper flakes
1/4 teaspoon ground cloves
1/4 teaspoon dried leaf thyme
3 large cloves garlic, quartered
8 sun-dried tomatoes
1 cup low-salt Italian tomatoes, chopped
1/2 cup fresh basil, chopped rough and loosely packed
   (leaves from a half-ounce bunch, or 11/2 teaspoons dried
   basil)

Rinse the lentils and stir into boiling water.

Add the remaining ingredients and bring to a low simmer for 40 minutes. While the lentils are simmering, soak the sun-dried tomatoes in just enough hot water to cover. When they are soft, cut them into 1/8-inch dice with a sharp knife. Do not process them, or they'll be lost in the stew.

After 40 minutes add the canned tomatoes, sun-dried tomatoes, and the basil.

Simmer for 10 minutes further. The lentils should be tender but still firm. If you cook them too long, they will explode and become thick and mushy. Try to achieve a tender, intact lentil in a soupy mixture. Taste the lentils for flavor; if your spices are older, you may need to add a pinch more thyme, cloves, or cayenne pepper. These flavors should not overpower one another or the lentils, but should each be present.

When the lentils are ready to serve, stir in the fresh basil.

SERVES 12

3/4 cup per serving

	Fat (g)	Cholesterol (g)	Sodium (mg)	Calories
Total Recipe	7.2	0	421.2	2196
Per Portion	.6	0	35.1	183

Chicken Stewed with Wine and Vegetables

This stew is akin to others like it, but it has the added nutrients of vegetables and potatoes. The carrots and parsley add beta-carotene.

chicken parts (3 split breast halves and 6 thighs)
3 tablespoons flour
1 medium onion, cut in 3/4-inch pieces
3 teaspoons fresh minced garlic
3 carrots, cut into thirds with the thick portion split
1 cup Ariél brand dealcoholized premium dry white wine
4 cups Low-Sodium Chicken Stock (see page 88)
1/2 teaspoon dried leaf thyme
1/2 teaspoon freshly ground black pepper
1/2 bay leaf
2 tablespoons fresh parsley
2 new potatoes, cut into 1-inch pieces
6 teaspoons freshly grated Parmesan cheese, optional

Preheat the oven to 350° F. Trim the chicken of all visible fat and skin.

Heat a heavy, nonstick skillet over medium-high heat. Sear the chicken, a few pieces at a time, until golden brown. Remove the chicken to a baking dish and sprinkle with the flour. Add the potatoes.

In the same pan, sauté the onion for 3–5 minutes. Add the garlic and sauté for 1 minute longer, being careful not to brown it.

Add the carrots and the wine. Bring to a simmer and cook to reduce the wine by half.

Add the chicken stock, thyme, pepper, and bay leaf. Pour over the meat and potatoes. Make sure all vegetables and meat are covered by liquid.

Cover the dish and bake in a 350°F oven for 1¼ hours, or until both the chicken and the vegetables are tender.

Remove and discard the bay leaf. If desired, serve with Parmesan cheese dusted over the top.

SERVES 6

	Fat (g)	Cholesterol (g)	Sodium (mg)	Calories
Total Recipe	55.8	535.2	1074	2880
Per Portion	9.3	89.2	179	480

Winter Stew

This is a robust stew and the turnips give it a special flavor, piqued by the Parmesan cheese and wine. It has the nutritional power of the winter root vegetables, including the beta-carotene of carrots, and is low in fat and sodium.

2 cups chopped leeks, cut into ¾-inch pieces
2 pounds lean bottom round roast of beef, trimmed of
     visible fat and cut into ¾-inch cubes
3 tablespoons flour
1½ cups Ariél brand dealcoholized premium red wine
2 cups onion, cut into ¾-inch pieces
1 cup celery, cut into ¾-inch pieces
1 cup thinly sliced carrots
½ pound turnips, cut into ¾-inch pieces
2 tablespoons fresh chopped garlic
½ teaspoon freshly ground black pepper
½ teaspoon dried leaf thyme
1 teaspoon dried rosemary
1 bay leaf
1/16 teaspoon ground clove, about 1 pinch
3 cups Low-Sodium Chicken Stock (see page 88)
4 teaspoons freshly grated Parmesan cheese

To prepare the leeks, split up the middle in quarters, leaving the stems intact. Hold the leeks under running water until all sand and debris are gone. Remove the darkest green portion before slicing.

Sprinkle the meat with the pepper and sauté in a heavy, nonstick skillet over medium-high heat. Do this a handful at a time to brown the meat; too much meat will reduce the temperature and it won't brown. Remove to a large baking dish and toss evenly with the flour.

Pour off any fat from the skillet. Add the wine and simmer to reduce by at least one-half. Add the reduced wine, vegetables, garlic, pepper, and herbs to the meat.

Add stock to barely cover the ingredients.

Preheat the oven to 350° F and cook covered for about 1½ hours or until the meat is very tender. Stir after one hour, making sure all ingredients are covered with liquid. Before serving, remove and discard bay leaf. Serve with a dusting of Parmesan cheese.

SERVES 8

1 cup per serving

	Fat (g)	Cholesterol (g)	Sodium (mg)	Calories
Total Recipe	51.2	680	798.4	2794.4
Per Portion	6.4	85	99.8	349.3

Peppered Yam Fries

These yams offer a satisfying and flavor-packed alternative to roasted white potatoes and even to French fries. Sprinkle them with a little malt or cider vinegar for the effect of English chips; their sweetness is a good backdrop for a hint of vinegar. The yams provide beta-carotene, and the olive oil is a good source of monounsaturated fat. Try them as a snack or with roasted meats or fish.

> 1 pound yams, washed, ends removed, and cut into finger-size pieces
> 1 1/2 teaspoons cracked black pepper
> 1 tablespoon extra virgin olive oil
> vegetable oil spray

Toss the yams with olive oil and then pepper.

Spray a baking sheet with vegetable oil spray and roast the yams in a pre-heated 375° F oven for 40–45 minutes. Turn the yams over halfway through the roasting.

SERVES 4

	Fat (g)	Cholesterol (g)	Sodium (mg)	Calories
Total Recipe	14	0	25.2	444
Per Portion	3.5	0	6.3	111

Roasted New Potatoes with Rosemary

These potatoes don't need sour cream or salt. They are a satisfying and robust way to serve potatoes with any roasted meat, fish, or hot sandwich.

> 8 new potatoes
> 1 tablespoon extra virgin olive oil
> 2 tablespoons chopped fresh rosemary, or 1 tablespoon dried
> 2 cloves fresh minced garlic

Wash and cut the potatoes in half.

Toss the potatoes with the oil and then the garlic and rosemary.

Preheat the oven to 375° F. Roast the potatoes for about 45 minutes, or until tender on the inside and crisp on the outside. A very sharp paring knife should be able to slip out easily after insertion.

SERVES 4

3/4 cup per serving

	Fat (g)	Cholesterol (g)	Sodium (mg)	Calories
Total Recipe	14.8	0	28.4	472
Per Portion	3.7	0	7.1	118

Baby Bliss Potatoes with Parsley

Potatoes are often the victim of fatty sauces, butter, or sour cream. This needn't happen since they are extremely low in fat, sodium, and calories in their natural state. This preparation doesn't ruin that record and is at once simple and comforting. Serve these potatoes alone or with "Sour Cream" Sauce (page 159).

2 pounds small new potatoes
3 tablespoons chopped fresh parsley

Wash the potatoes and make sure they are of equal size. If not, cut the largest ones in half.

Either steam the potatoes or boil them. They are done when a sharp knife slips out easily after insertion.

Drain them and keep covered until serving. Serve tossed with parsley.

SERVES 6

	Fat (g)	Cholesterol (g)	Sodium (mg)	Calories
Total Recipe	.3	0	22.2	270.6
Per Portion	trace	0	3.7	45.1

— Potato and Celery Root — Purée

With the addition of celery root (celeriac) to whipped potatoes, there is little need for ladles of gravy or butter. Serve these potatoes with any roasted meat or instead of mashed potatoes. They are low in sodium, fat, and calories, but you wouldn't know it by tasting them.

1 pound russet potatoes (or similar), peeled and cut into 1/2-inch cubes
3/4–1 pound celery root, trimmed and cut into 1/2-inch cubes
1/2 cup nonfat plain yogurt
1/16 teaspoon cayenne pepper (about 1 large pinch)
1/8 teaspoon freshly grated nutmeg (or more, if not freshly grated)

When preparing the celery root remove all of the outer skin, which is tough and dark brown. Keep both the potato and celery root pieces under water after they are cut into pieces, to keep them from turning brown.

Place the celery root in a medium-sized, heavy saucepan and put the potato on top. Add 1/2-inch water to the pan. Cover the pan and bring water to a boil.

Steam the vegetables for about 12 minutes, or until both are cooked and tender. When they are soft, remove the lid and cook until the water evaporates.

Using a ricer or mixer, purée the vegetables with the spices and yogurt and serve immediately. Do not overprocess. The mixture will toughen. If you must reheat before serving, do so at a low temperature so the yogurt won't separate.

SERVES 6

	Fat (g)	Cholesterol (g)	Sodium (mg)	Calories
Total Recipe	1.8	0	413.4	450
Per Portion	.3	0	68.9	75

Roasted Shallots

Roasted shallots make a robust accompaniment to any roasted meat. They are also delicious spread on toasted bread and on pizza. They can accompany any herb-roasted meat without the need for a rich and fatty sauce.

8 shallots

Peel and split the shallots in half, creating equal-sized pieces.

Roast the shallots on a baking sheet in a 375° F oven for about 50 minutes, depending on the size. They should be soft with a golden caramel color on the surface.

SERVES 4
4 shallot halves per serving

	Fat (g)	Cholesterol (g)	Sodium (mg)	Calories
Total Recipe	0	0	4	12
Per Portion	0	0	1	3

Sugar Snap Peas with Red Onion and Cilantro

This recipe is low in sodium, fat, and calories and is a simple and zesty way to enjoy fresh sugar snap peas.

3/4 pound sugar snap peas, or fresh snow peas
1 cup red onion, sliced finely (about 1 medium red onion)
1 tablespoon safflower, sunflower, corn, canola, or light olive oil
2 teaspoons fresh minced garlic
1/4 cup rice vinegar
3 tablespoons chopped fresh cilantro

Pick the ends from the sugar snap peas (or snow peas) while pulling off as much of the string that runs along the underside of the pod as will come free.

In a large, heavy, nonstick skillet or wok, heat the oil until hot.

Add the onion and sauté for 1–2 minutes or until it begins to wilt.

Then add the peas and cook for about 1 minute stirring occasionally. The pan should remain hot.

Add the minced garlic to the pan, wait a few seconds, and toss.

Stir in the vinegar and simmer until all the liquid has evaporated.

Add the cilantro, toss, and serve.

SERVES 4

3/4 cup per serving

	Fat (g)	Cholesterol (g)	Sodium (mg)	Calories
Total Recipe	14	0	34	266
Per Portion	3.5	0	8.5	66.5

Green Beans with Garlic and Balsamic Vinegar

Here's a green bean dish with lots of flavor but little fat and sodium. Try it with presteamed, dark green, leafy vegetables, such as collard greens and kale.

1 pound green beans
2 tablespoons extra virgin olive oil
1 teaspoon fresh minced garlic
1/2 teaspoon freshly ground black pepper
2 tablespoons balsamic vinegar

Wash and trim the beans. Steam them until tender but not mushy, or cook them in boiling water for 3–4 minutes. Remove them from the heat and run them under cold water to stop the cooking.

Just before serving, sauté the garlic in the olive oil for about 2 minutes; do not brown.

Add the beans and toss while cooking, about 3 minutes.

Add the pepper and balsamic vinegar and cook until the vinegar is almost gone.

SERVES 5

	Fat (g)	Cholesterol (g)	Sodium (mg)	Calories
Total Recipe	27.5	0	16.5	331.5
Per Portion	5.5	0	3.3	66.3

Bok Choy with Ginger and Apples

This version of Chinese cabbage is sweet and full of the power of ginger. It can serve four as a side dish or two for a full meal with rice.

vegetable oil spray
1/4 cup onion, finely sliced (about 1/4 medium onion)
2 teaspoons grated fresh ginger
2 cups Granny Smith apple pieces, sliced 1/4-inch thick
2 tablespoons rice vinegar
3 cups bok choy, 1/2-inch slices at an angle
2 tablespoons Ariél brand dealcoholized premium dry white wine
1/8 teaspoon white pepper

Heat a large, heavy, nonstick skillet or wok to medium-high, spray it with vegetable spray, and add the onion and ginger. Stir them, being careful that the ginger doesn't stick and burn. It is important that the ginger cooks, so that it retains its flavor without the heat. Cook about 2 minutes.

Add the apple and cook for about 2 minutes, or until the pieces begin to turn golden brown. If the pan loses heat, water will collect and the apples won't brown. Keep the pan hot.

Add the vinegar and allow it to reduce until it has completely evaporated. Quickly add the cabbage and stir.

Reduce the heat to medium and cover the pan for 1–2 minutes, or until the cabbage starts to wilt.

Add the wine, cover the pan, and cook for 2 more minutes.

Remove the cover, stir in the pepper, and let the wine and other liquids evaporate. Serve right away.

SERVES 4
3/4 cup per serving

	Fat (g)	Cholesterol (g)	Sodium (mg)	Calories
Total Recipe	.8	0	145.2	196.4
Per Portion	.2	0	36.3	49.1

Celery Cabbage with Ginger and Red Grapes

This cabbage dish can be served as a side dish or with rice as a vegetarian main course. It has all the nutrients of cabbage and is low in fat, calories, and sodium.

> 1 teaspoon sesame oil
> 1 teaspoon safflower, corn, canola, or light olive oil
> 6 cups celery cabbage, sliced 1/3-inch thick
> 3 scallions, dark green part removed, in 1-inch slivers
> 2 teaspoons minced or grated fresh ginger root
> 1/2 teaspoon freshly ground black pepper
> 1 teaspoon sugar
> 1/4 cup rice vinegar
> 1/2 cup red seedless grapes, cut in half
> 2 teaspoons unsalted, roasted peanuts

In a large, heavy, nonstick skillet or wok, heat the two oils to medium-high.

Sauté the scallions and ginger for 1–2 minutes, keeping the ginger from browning too much.

Add the cabbage and sauté 2 minutes further, or until it just begins to wilt.

Sprinkle the cabbage with the pepper, sugar, and vinegar, and cook to reduce the vinegar. Meanwhile, chop the peanuts very fine or grind them in the food processor fitted with a metal blade.

Add the grapes to the cabbage and toss. Serve with the ground peanuts sprinkled on top.

SERVES 4

	Fat (g)	Cholesterol (g)	Sodium (mg)	Calories
Total Recipe	15.6	0	280	289.6
Per Portion	3.9	0	70	72.4

Braised Sweet and Sour Cabbage

This a very rich and flavorful cabbage. Extremely low in sodium and fat, it provides the nutrients of the Cruciferous family. Try it for people who think they don't like cabbage.

4 cups shredded Savoy cabbage
1 cup onions, sliced very fine (about 1 medium onion)
1 tablespoon extra virgin olive oil
¼ cup plus 1 tablespoon sherry wine vinegar or balsamic
  vinegar
¼ cup Low-Sodium Chicken Stock (see page 88)
2 tablespoons sugar
½ teaspoon cracked black pepper
½ teaspoon dry mustard

Heat a large, heavy, nonstick skillet over medium-high heat. Divide the cabbage into three parts and sauté each portion in ⅓ of the olive oil, about 2–3 minutes each. The edges should just begin to turn dark, and the pan should be hot enough so that water does not build up. Remove each part to a platter or bowl when done, and let the pan get hot again.

Sauté the onions in the same fashion, but let them brown well and remove.

Add ¼ cup sherry vinegar, stock, sugar, pepper, and mustard. Reduce by half, stirring up the brown bits from the pan.

Return the cabbage and onion to the pan and toss together with the broth. Cover the pan and reduce the heat to medium. Cook for about 10 minutes longer; any remaining liquid should disappear.

Sprinkle the cabbage with 1 tablespoon sherry vinegar and toss. Serve hot or cold.

SERVES 4

¾ cup per serving

	Fat (g)	Cholesterol (g)	Sodium (mg)	Calories
Total Recipe	15.2	0	83.2	366
Per Portion	3.8	0	20.8	91.5

Golden Cauliflower

This simple preparation is for those who think they don't like cauliflower without a flood of butter or cheese. It has eye appeal without a fatty sauce smothering the wonderful taste of the cauliflower. Also try adding a pinch of curry powder.

1 pound cauliflower, cut into florets (1 small cauliflower)
1/16 teaspoon ground turmeric (about one large pinch)

Drop the florets into 1/3 inch of boiling water. Try to place the stalk sides down, if possible.

Cover and simmer for 2–3 minutes or until the stem is pliable.

Drain the cauliflower, dust it with turmeric, and let it rest, covered, for 5 minutes.

SERVES 4
3/4 cup per serving

	Fat (g)	Cholesterol (g)	Sodium (mg)	Calories
Total Recipe	1.6	0	28.4	60
Per Portion	.4	0	7.1	15

Cauliflower with Walnuts and Parmesan

Most gratins use cream and cheese. This one is lower in fat, sodium, and calories but is just as rich. Serve it with other colorful dishes, since cauliflower is on the pale side.

1 medium cauliflower, stem removed and cut into florets
2 tablespoons Thickest Yogurt (page 88)
2 tablespoons minced walnuts
4 tablespoons freshly grated Parmesan cheese

Steam the cauliflower florets until slightly soft. Remove from the heat.

Chop or mash the warm cauliflower and fold in the yogurt. Gently press the mixture into a small baking dish and sprinkle with the walnuts and then the cheese.

Broil for 2–3 minutes until the top is golden brown.

SERVES 5

	Fat (g)	Cholesterol (g)	Sodium (mg)	Calories
Total Recipe	16.5	4.4	600	297.2
Per Portion	3.3	2.2	120	59.4

—— Spaghetti Squash with —— Parsley and Sweet Pepper

Spaghetti squash is a fresh-tasting variation on a pasta side dish. An added bonus: most winter squashes are high in beta-carotene.

1¼ pound spaghetti squash (about ½ medium squash)
1 teaspoon extra virgin olive oil
½ teaspoon cracked black pepper
3 tablespoons chopped fresh parsley
¼ cup sweet red pepper, very finely diced (about ⅓ of a
**   medium pepper)**

Wash the squash, cut off its stem, and cut it lengthwise in half.

Place the squash cut side down in a steamer basket and steam it for about 15 minutes, or until its strands pull away from the skin easily with a fork. The strands should be intact; cooking too long turns them mushy.

In a medium, heavy nonstick skillet, heat the olive oil over medium-high heat. When the oil is hot, add the pepper. When the pepper aroma is rich, add the squash and remaining ingredients and cook until fully heated. Serve hot.

SERVES 4

½ cup per serving

	Fat (g)	Cholesterol (g)	Sodium (mg)	Calories
Total Recipe	7	0	7.4	208.4
Per Portion	1.8	0	1.9	52.1

Spaghetti Squash with Basil

Another variation on spaghetti squash, this one offers the same beta-carotene with the slightly anise flavor of basil and shallots. This dish is extremely low in calories, sodium, and fat.

1¼ pounds spaghetti squash (about ½ medium squash)
1 teaspoon extra virgin olive oil
4 tablespoons finely chopped shallots
4 teaspoons balsamic vinegar
¹/₁₆ teaspoon white pepper (about 1 large pinch)
3 tablespoons very thinly sliced fresh basil leaves

Wash the squash, remove its stem, and cut in half.

Place the squash cut side down in a steamer basket and steam it for about 15 minutes, or until its strands pull away from the skin easily with a fork. The strands should be intact; cooking too long turns them mushy.

Heat the olive oil in a medium, heavy, nonstick skillet over medium-high heat. Add the shallots and sauté for about 5 minutes until the edges start to brown.

Add half the balsamic vinegar and reduce until almost dry.

Right away, stir in the squash and the basil. Drizzle with the remaining vinegar, add the white pepper, and toss. Serve hot or cold.

SERVES 4
½ cup per serving

	Fat (g)	Cholesterol (g)	Sodium (mg)	Calories
Total Recipe	6.9	0	8	213.6
Per Portion	1.7	0	2	53.4

— Acorn Squash with Mace —

Acorn squash has all the power of beta-carotene, and this recipe is low in sodium, calories, and fat. The sweetness of the squash is complemented by a hint of mace and ginger.

2 medium acorn squash (makes 2 cups cooked squash)
2 teaspoons extra virgin olive oil
1/2 teaspoon ground mace
1 teaspoon dry ginger
1/2 cup homemade Low Sodium Chicken Stock (page 88)

Wash the squash, remove the stems, and cut in half lengthwise. Remove the seeds and strands from the middle with a fork and steam the squash open side down for about 15 minutes; or, steam for 7 minutes and bake for an additional 10 minutes in a 350° F oven. Scrape the squash away from its skin with a large spoon, and mash or chop it.

In a large, heavy, nonstick skillet, heat the oil over medium-high heat. Add the squash and sprinkle with the mace and ginger. Turn the squash periodically.

As it gets dry, add the stock. Allow the stock to reduce by half and serve hot.

SERVES 4

1/2 cup per serving

	Fat (g)	Cholesterol (g)	Sodium (mg)	Calories
Total Recipe	14	0	4.9	271.6
Per Portion	3.5	0	1.23	67.9

Broccoli with Pine Nuts and Raisins

Broccoli is a member of the Cruciferous family, and this recipe offers a lot of flavor. You might want to try the preparation with any dark green, leafy vegetable, such as collard greens or mustard greens. The nuts and raisins add a hint of sweetness to the sweet and sour vinegar.

1 pound broccoli
1 teaspoon extra virgin olive oil
1/4 cup golden raisins
1/4 cup balsamic vinegar
2 tablespoons pine nuts, roasted
1 teaspoon coarse freshly ground black pepper

Wash and trim the broccoli by cutting up from the stems, separating the florets. The stem portions of each piece should be fairly equal to the others.

Steam the broccoli for about 3 minutes with the stems closest to the water. The broccoli should be tender but still firm.

Over medium-high heat, heat the olive oil in a large, heavy, nonstick skillet. Add the broccoli and raisins and sauté for about 3 minutes. The pan should NOT be so hot as to brown the broccoli.

Add the balsamic vinegar and let it reduce until it is a syrup. Add the pepper and toss with the nuts.

SERVES 4

	Fat (g)	Cholesterol (g)	Sodium (mg)	Calories
Total Recipe	19.6	0	54.4	347.6
Per Portion	4.9	0	13.6	86.9

— Curried Butternut Squash —

Butternut squash, like the other winter squashes, is high in beta-carotene and naturally low in sodium, fat, and calories. But because butternut is so naturally sweet, it needs little added to it.

**3 pounds butternut squash, skinned, seeded, and cut into
3/4-inch cubes
2 teaspoons curry powder
1/16 teaspoon cayenne pepper (about 1 large pinch)
1/2 cup Low-Sodium Chicken Stock (see page 88)
1/2 cup nonfat plain yogurt**

Cook the squash covered for about 10 minutes in a medium-sized saucepan with the chicken stock, which should rise about 1 inch in the pan. Stir after 5 minutes.

Remove the lid from the pan. If the squash is tender, let the liquid evaporate. If not, cook covered for a few more minutes.

Purée or whip the squash with the spices and yogurt and serve immediately. If you must reheat the squash, do so at a low temperature to keep the yogurt from separating.

SERVES 4

1/2 cup per serving

	Fat (g)	Cholesterol (g)	Sodium (mg)	Calories
Total Recipe	3.6	0	124	246.8
Per Portion	.9	0	31	61.7

Carrots with Orange and Sage

This carrot dish is just as welcome with a holiday roast as it is with a lighter fish entrée like Tuna with Avocado Papaya Relish (page 182).

3/4 pound thin or baby carrots, steamed
3/4 cup fresh squeezed orange juice
2 teaspoons orange zest, minced, with no white pulp
1 tablespoon honey
3/4 cup Low-Sodium Chicken Stock (see page 88)
4 sage leaves, sliced wafer-thin (or 1/4 teaspoon dried sage
   leaves)

The carrots should be equal-sized or cut into equal-sized pieces about 3 inches in length. Steam the carrots until they are cooked but slightly firm.

In a medium-sized saucepan, cover the steamed carrots with the orange juice, orange zest, honey, and chicken stock.

Simmer the carrots over medium heat, letting the carrots cook while the liquid thickens to form a glaze that will coat the carrots.

Serve with fresh sage (or dried) sprinkled over the top.

SERVES 4

	Fat (g)	Cholesterol (g)	Sodium (mg)	Calories
Total Recipe	2.28	0	154.8	278.4
Per Portion	.57	0	38.7	69.6

Gingered Carrots

These carrots are loaded with beta-carotene and the sweetness of ginger and pineapple. The recipe is very low in fat, calories, and sodium.

3/4 pound thin or baby carrots, peeled
pineapple juice to cover
1 1/2 teaspoons grated fresh ginger root
1 teaspoon unsalted margarine

Cut the carrots into 3-inch pieces. Split the larger pieces if they are oversized compared to the others. Uniformly sized carrots will cook evenly. Layer the carrots in a pan with the larger carrots on the bottom.

Cover with the juice and ginger and bring to a simmer. Cook for 10–15 minutes or until tender.

Remove the carrots and continue cooking the sauce until it is reduced to a syrup. Blend the margarine into the syrup; add the carrots and stir to coat.

SERVES 4

	Fat (g)	Cholesterol (g)	Sodium (mg)	Calories
Total Recipe	2.8	0	78	251.6
Per Portion	.7	0	19.5	62.9

Simply Mushrooms

These mushrooms are great for flavoring a side dish, with roasted meats, on sandwiches, as a stuffing in breads, or stirred into a soup.

1/2 fresh pound mushrooms, 1/4-inch sliced
1/2 cup Ariél brand dealcoholized premium dry white wine
1/2 cup Low-Sodium Chicken Stock (see page 88)
1/8 teaspoon dried thyme leaves
1/8 teaspoon freshly ground black pepper

Heat a large, heavy, nonstick skillet over medium-high heat. Spray it with vegetable spray and add the mushrooms. Sauté for about 4 minutes, stirring to cook both sides. Remove them to a dish and let them rest. Drain the juices and reserve.

Return the mushrooms to the pan and cook over medium-high heat until they start to brown. Add the wine and simmer uncovered until almost all the liquid has evaporated. (If you like your mushrooms al dente, remove them before the wine starts to reduce and add them after the next step.)

Add the chicken stock, mushroom juices, thyme, and pepper and cook until syrupy. If you are using them as a sandwich spread, chop them coarsely.

SERVES 4
1/3 cup per serving

	Fat (g)	Cholesterol (g)	Sodium (mg)	Calories
Total Recipe	1.2	0	47.2	122.4
Per Portion	.3	0	11.8	30.6

Brussels Sprouts with Caraway

Brussels sprouts are in the Cruciferous family, and this recipe is low in fat and sodium. It has a lot of flavor and, for people who think they don't like brussels sprouts, this would be a good risk. Balsamic vinegar is less acidic and sweeter than regular wine vinegar; it offers great flavor without the need for added salt. It is available in gourmet markets if your local supermarket doesn't carry it.

1 pound brussels sprouts
1½ teaspoons fresh minced garlic
2 teaspoons extra virgin olive oil
2 teaspoons caraway seeds
2 teaspoons balsamic vinegar

Trim any brown leaves from the brussels sprouts and trim the ends. Make a shallow cross in the stem, which allows them to cook thoroughly.

Put the brussels sprouts in a medium, heavy, nonstick saucepan with a tightly fitting lid. The sprouts should fit rather tightly in the bottom of the pan, without a steaming basket. Add ¼ inch of water. Let the stems rest in the water and cover the pan tightly. Cook them for 4–5 minutes; the stems will cook while the leaves steam. They should be cooked and pliable, but not soft. Remove them from the heat and drain.

Just before serving, heat the olive oil and garlic in a medium-sized, heavy, nonstick skillet over medium-high heat. Do not let the garlic brown.

When the garlic emits its aroma and the pan is hot, add the brussels sprouts and caraway seeds. The brussels sprouts will brown very lightly and the caraway will release its aroma. Stir them occasionally, cooking for 3–4 minutes.

Add the balsamic vinegar and toss the sprouts. Serve when the vinegar is reduced to a syrup and has glazed the sprouts.

SERVES 4

	Fat (g)	Cholesterol (g)	Sodium (mg)	Calories
Total Recipe	9.8	0	46.4	176.4
Per Portion	2.5	0	11.6	44.1

Barbecue Sauce

This sauce is a low-sodium way to add zing to roasted meats. Barbe-cued meats are usually fatty and salty. Using low-fat meats and this sauce, you can still have that summer treat. This sauce is rather thick and can be thinned, if you wish, with a little water.

vegetable oil spray
1 cup chopped onion (about 1 medium onion)
1 tablespoon chopped fresh garlic
1/4 cup red wine vinegar
8 ounces no-salt tomato sauce
1 tablespoon low-salt Worcestershire sauce
1/2 teaspoon red pepper flakes
1 teaspoon no-salt Dijon mustard (or regular variety)
4 sun-dried tomato halves
1 tablespoon molasses
1 tablespoon honey

Heat a heavy saucepan over medium-high heat and spray it with veg-etable oil spray. Add the onion. Reduce the heat and let the onion brown slowly; allow it to caramelize but not to burn.

Add the garlic and vinegar and scrape up the brown particles from the bottom of the pan. Let the vinegar reduce to a syrup.

Add the remaining ingredients except the honey.

Cook on a low simmer for at least 40 minutes. Partially cover the pan to keep it from spattering.

Purée the sauce in a food processor and add the honey.

Keep refrigerated. Makes about 1 cup.

SERVES 18
1 tablespoon per serving

	Fat (g)	Cholesterol (g)	Sodium (mg)	Calories
Total Recipe	7.2	0	732	1089.6
Per Portion	.4	0	40.6	60.5

Hot Sauce

This hot sauce is a lot lower in sodium than most store-bought varieties and can come in handy for spicing up meats, vegetables, and rice. Use it as you would any other hot pepper sauce.

1/2 cup Barbecue Sauce (page 154)
1/2 cup red wine vinegar
1/2 cup water
1/4 teaspoon cayenne pepper, or to taste

Combine all of the ingredients and stir until well blended. Taste and adjust the cayenne pepper to your liking.

SERVES 52
1 teaspoon per serving

	Fat (g)	Cholesterol (g)	Sodium (mg)	Calories
Total Recipe	3.4	0	252	379.2
Per Portion	trace	0	4.6	7

Ketchup

This ketchup is much lower in sodium than the store-bought variety and has a rich flavor.

1/2 cup Barbecue Sauce (page 154)
1/2 cup water
1/2 cup low-sodium vegetable juice
1 teaspoon sugar

Place all of the ingredients in a small bowl and stir until well blended. If you like a thinner ketchup, add more water.

SERVES 18
1 tablespoon per serving

	Fat (g)	Cholesterol (g)	Sodium (mg)	Calories
Total Recipe	2.4	0	266.5	393.2
Per Portion	0	0	14.8	21.8

Mustard Sauce

This sauce can be served over both cold and steaming hot vegetables or with meats. It has a rich mustard flavor without much fat or added sodium. If you can't find low-sodium Dijon mustard, use the regular variety and add 57 milligrams of sodium per serving.

1/2 cup Thickest Yogurt (page 88)
2 teaspoons minced onion
2 tablespoons no-salt Dijon mustard
1 teaspoon champagne or tarragon vinegar
1/4 teaspoon coarse black pepper

Combine all the ingredients.

Serve at room temperature for hot foods.

SERVES 6

	Fat (g)	Cholesterol (g)	Sodium (mg)	Calories
Total Recipe	7.2	0	370.8	222
Per Portion	1.2	0	61.8	37

Pizza Sauce

This pizza sauce lacks the sodium of most, is very low in fat, and can help turn pizza into a healthy treat that tastes like it should. This sauce will make one pizza.

2 teaspoons extra virgin olive oil
1/4 cup finely chopped onion
4 teaspoons minced fresh garlic, or more to taste
1/2 teaspoon dried oregano
1/2 teaspoon dried basil
1/4 teaspoon cayenne pepper
8 ounces no-salt tomato sauce
1/2 teaspoon sugar

Heat the olive oil in a small, heavy, nonaluminum saucepan over medium-high heat. Sauté the onion and garlic for 2–3 minutes or until they start to turn clear.

Add the herbs, spices, and tomato sauce and simmer for about 10 minutes, partially covering the pan to keep the sauce from spattering.

Stir in the sugar to taste.

SERVES 4

	Fat (g)	Cholesterol (g)	Sodium (mg)	Calories
Total Recipe	8.8	0	208.8	319.6
Per Portion	2.2	0	52.2	79.9

— Yogurt with Mint, Chili, — and Onion

This is a nonfat, low-sodium, and low-calorie accompaniment for any curried dish. It adds flavor, tartness, and a little heat. Try it with Curried Black Beans (page 109).

1 cup nonfat plain yogurt
1/8 teaspoon ground cayenne pepper
2 tablespoons fresh chopped mint
2 tablespoons fresh chopped cilantro
2 tablespoons minced onion
1/2 teaspoon minced jalapeño

Stir all ingredients together and chill for 1 hour before serving.

Serve in a side dish or spooned on top of the curried dish.

SERVES 8

	Fat (g)	Cholesterol (g)	Sodium (mg)	Calories
Total Recipe	trace	0	224.8	172
Per Portion	trace	0	28.1	21.5

Dill Sauce

This nonfat and low-sodium sauce is a subtle complement to poached fish, especially salmon. Serve your fish with a simple, cool salad, like Cucumber Salad with Dill (page 121).

> 2 tablespoons minced onion
> 2 tablespoons Ariél brand dealcoholized premium dry white wine
> 1 cup nonfat plain yogurt
> 1/4 teaspoon freshly ground black pepper
> 2 tablespoons fresh dill (or 1 1/2 teaspoons dry dill)
> 1/16 teaspoon cayenne pepper, or to taste

In a small, nonstick skillet or pan, sauté the onion until clear. Do not brown.

Add the wine and reduce until it thickens to resemble a syrup. Remove from the heat and let cool.

Just before serving, add the remaining ingredients and blend. Warm the sauce slowly over low heat. Do not let the sauce approach boiling or it will separate.

Serve with hot fish. Or don't reheat the sauce and serve it chilled with poached, chilled fish.

SERVES 6

	Fat (g)	Cholesterol (g)	Sodium (mg)	Calories
Total Recipe	0	0	168	150
Per Portion	0	0	28	25

"Sour Cream" Sauce

This sauce is low in fat and sodium and is a great way to adorn your baked potatoes, vegetables, or sandwiches. You'll wonder where all the flavor comes from.

1 tablespoon finely minced onion
1 cup low-fat plain yogurt
1/8 teaspoon freshly ground black pepper
chopped fresh chives (optional)

Stir the ingredients together and refrigerate for at least 1 hour before serving to release the flavors.

SERVES 6
2 tablespoons per serving

	Fat (g)	Cholesterol (g)	Sodium (mg)	Calories
Total Recipe	4	12	162	150
Per Portion	.6	2	27	25

——— Horseradish Sauce ———

This sauce is for the horseradish lover. It is a low-fat, low-sodium accompaniment for roast beef, hot or cold.

1 tablespoon prepared horseradish, or to taste
1 tablespoon finely minced onion
1 cup low-fat plain yogurt
1/8 teaspoon freshly ground black pepper

In a small bowl, stir the ingredients together. Refrigerate for at least 1 hour before serving to release the flavors.
SERVES 6

	Fat (g)	Cholesterol (g)	Sodium (mg)	Calories
Total Recipe	4	12	246	186
Per Portion	.6	2	41	31

— Tomato Rosemary Sauce —

This is a basic tomato sauce without added salt or sugar. The flavor of the carrot reduces the need for salt and sugar. Serve it with pasta, fish, or veal.

2 tablespoons extra virgin olive oil
1 medium onion, chopped
2 tablespoons plus 1/2 teaspoon chopped fresh garlic
11/4 teaspoons fennel seed
1/2 teaspoon red pepper flakes
1 28-ounce can no-salt Italian tomatoes, roughly chopped
11/2 cups of the juice from canned tomatoes
1 medium carrot, cut lengthwise into 1/8-inch strips
2 bay leaves
1/2 teaspoon dried leaf thyme
1 teaspoon dried rosemary

Heat the olive oil in a heavy, nonaluminum skillet over medium-high heat. Sauté the onion and 2 tablespoons of the garlic until partly clear, being careful not to brown.

Add fennel seed and red pepper flakes and sauté 3 minutes uncovered to evoke their aroma.

Add remaining ingredients and simmer for 30 minutes or until the carrot is tender.

Remove from the heat. Mince the remaining 1/2 teaspoon garlic until very fine, stir into the sauce, and let rest for 10 minutes. Meanwhile, remove and discard bay leaf. Place the carrot and 1/2 cup of the sauce in the blender or a food processor fitted with a metal blade and purée until smooth. Stir the puréed carrot into the sauce.

SERVES 8

	Fat (g)	Cholesterol (g)	Sodium (mg)	Calories
Total Recipe	28	0	541.6	1840
Per Portion	3.5	0	67.7	230

—— Wild Mushroom Sauce ——

This sauce is rich and flavorful. The veal stock provides a thick sauce without the added fat in most gravies. Serve it with veal or beef, like Broiled Veal Flank with Rosemary and Garlic (page 200).

**1/4 pound fresh wild mushrooms, portobello and/or shiitake
vegetable oil spray
1 teaspoon unsalted margarine
3 tablespoons finely chopped shallots
1/2 cup Ariél brand dealcoholized premium dry white wine
1/4 teaspoon dried leaf thyme
1/4 bay leaf
2 cups rich Veal Stock (see page 91)**

Clean the mushrooms; remove, chop, and set aside the stems. Slice the mushroom tops in 1/4-inch slices.

Heat a large, heavy skillet over medium-high heat. Spray the hot pan with vegetable oil spray and sauté or stir-fry the mushrooms for 5–7 minutes or until the edges start to wilt. Remove immediately to a plate and cool.

Heat the margarine in a heavy saucepan over medium-high heat. Sauté the shallots until translucent. Add the wine and simmer, reducing the wine to a syrup. (If the stock is not meaty and rich, add 3 tablespoons chopped onion, 2 tablespoons minced carrot, and 1 tablespoon minced celery.)

Add the herbs, mushroom stems, stock, and any mushroom drippings that have accumulated. Cook at a simmer and do not stir the sauce often. Reduce about 20 minutes until ¼ of the volume remains and the sauce has thickened.

Remove and discard bay leaf. Strain the sauce in a large sieve, pressing the vegetables lightly, and return it to the pan, adding the mushrooms. Serve hot.

SERVES 6

	Fat (g)	Cholesterol (g)	Sodium (mg)	Calories
Total Recipe	4.8	0	145.8	195
Per Portion	.8	0	24.3	32.5

Raspberry Sauce

This is a brown sauce and provides the richness of a gravy without the fat. It is a "sweet and sour" accompaniment to veal, pork, or beef.

3 tablespoons chopped shallots
1 teaspoon unsalted margarine
¼ cup raspberry vinegar
½ cup fresh sweet raspberries
1/16 teaspoon ground white pepper (about 1 pinch)
¼ teaspoon dried leaf thyme
¼ bay leaf
2 cups rich Veal Stock (see page 91)

In a saucepan sauté the shallots in the margarine until translucent. Add the vinegar and reduce to a syrup. (If the stock is not meaty and rich, add 3 tablespoons chopped onion, 2 tablespoons minced carrot, and 1 tablespoon minced celery.)

Add the herbs, stock, and half of the raspberries. Cook the sauce at a simmer; do not boil or stir it often. Reduce about 20 minutes until ¼ of the volume remains and the sauce has thickened.

Remove and discard bay leaf. Strain the sauce, pressing the raspberries into the sieve. Return the sauce to the pan with the remainder of the raspberries. Serve hot.

SERVES 6

	Fat (g)	Cholesterol (g)	Sodium (mg)	Calories
Total Recipe	4.8	0	133.8	123
Per Portion	.8	0	22.3	20.5

– Roasted Red Pepper Relish –

This relish is as intense in flavor as it is rich in nutrients. It makes a delicious relish for broiled fish or meats. It also complements sandwiches made from sliced roasted meats.

1 large green pepper
1 large sweet red pepper
1 large yellow pepper
2 tablespoons minced shallots
1½ teaspoons minced garlic
¼ teaspoon dried leaf thyme
2 tablespoons extra virgin olive oil

Place the peppers on a baking sheet and broil 2 inches from the element, turning with tongs to allow all sides to blister and blacken. This takes about 10 minutes.

Put the peppers directly into a covered bowl and cool.

Heat the remaining ingredients in a small saucepan on low heat. Continue warming until they are translucent, about five minutes. Do not brown.

When cool enough to handle, peel the skins from the peppers, removing all seeds, trying not to rinse away the juices. Thinly slice the peppers, about ¼-inch wide. Toss with the oil mixture.

Serve at room temperature.

SERVES 6

	Fat (g)	Cholesterol (g)	Sodium (mg)	Calories
Total Recipe	28.2	0	10	306
Per Portion	4.7	0	2	51

- Pineapple Mustard Chutney -

Serve this nearly fat-free and low-sodium chutney with roasted chicken or pork. It is delicious with sautéed boneless chicken breasts as a hot salad or cold sandwich. Try it with a garnish of fresh sliced basil. If you can't find low-sodium Dijon mustard, use the regular variety and add 57 milligrams of sodium per serving.

3/4 cup canned pineapple pieces, unsweetened
2 tablespoons no-salt Dijon mustard
1 tablespoon honey

In a food processor fitted with a metal blade, process the pineapple until it is chopped into 1/8-inch pieces.

Add the Dijon mustard and honey and pulse the processor several times until well blended. If you prefer a hotter or sweeter chutney, add more mustard or honey.

SERVES 8

	Fat (g)	Cholesterol (g)	Sodium (mg)	Calories
Total Recipe	7.2	0	210.4	108
Per Portion	.9	0	26.3	13.5

- Mango and Melon Chutney -

This is a fresh chutney and works well with many spicy curried dishes since it is subtly cool and refreshing. It is also rich in beta-carotene and delicious served as is with fish and chicken. Try it with Southwestern Chicken (page 188) or with Curried Black Beans (page 109). If for some reason you can't find mangos, you can use ripe peaches.

3/4 cup ripe and firm mango
1/2 teaspoon cracked black pepper
3/4 cup santa claus or honeydew melon
2 tablespoons purple bell pepper or sweet red pepper
2 teaspoons minced red onion
1 tablespoon rice vinegar
1 tablespoon Ariél brand dealcoholized premium white
**   Zinfandel wine**
2 teaspoons chopped fresh mint
1 tablespoon chopped fresh cilantro

Carefully cut the mango into uniformly shaped cubes, between 1/4 and 1/3 inch. Place in the serving bowl and sprinkle with the cracked black pepper. Cut the melon in the same fashion and place it next to the mango.

Create a fine dice of the purple pepper about 1/4-inch wide and add to the serving bowl, keeping the ingredients separate until the end. Mince the onion and add to the bowl.

Drizzle the vinegar and wine over all of the ingredients. Sprinkle the mint and cilantro over the fruit and fold the ingredients together with a few strokes.

Let the chutney rest for at least an hour in the refrigerator. It can be prepared several hours ahead of time.

SERVES 8

	Fat (g)	Cholesterol (g)	Sodium (mg)	Calories
Total Recipe	.8	0	19.2	109.6
Per Portion	.1	0	2.4	13.7

— Papaya and Citrus Relish —

This relish is great for baked or broiled fish and for warmed oysters on the half shell (see Warmed Oysters with Spinach and Papaya, page 184). Or try it with any medium-bodied fish. Since it makes a generous two cups of relish, you can use this recipe as a dip with sturdy lettuce leaves, like Radicchio. It is high in vitamin C and beta-carotene. For an accompaniment, try serving Gingered Rolls (page 225) with the meal.

1 ripe papaya
2 tablespoons black papaya seeds
1/2 cup freshly squeezed orange juice
1 tablespoon fresh lime juice
2 teaspoons minced shallots
1 jalapeño, deseeded and minced
minced zest of one lime
6 tablespoons chopped fresh cilantro

With a sharp knife make a very fine dice of the papaya, about 1/4-inch thick. The pieces should be uniform in size and shape.

To prepare the jalapeño pepper, wash the pepper and remove the stem portion. Slice the pepper lengthwise and remove the seeds under cold running water. Mince it with a very sharp knife and immediately wash your hands with soap and warm water.

In a medium serving bowl, gently fold all the ingredients together and let the relish rest in the refrigerator for at least one hour. Taste the relish; it should be slightly sweet from the orange juice and papaya. If your fruits aren't sweet, add sugar to taste. Remove to room temperature before serving.

SERVES 6

	Fat (g)	Cholesterol (g)	Sodium (mg)	Calories
Total Recipe	.6	0	17.4	217.8
Per Portion	.1	0	2.9	37.3

Black Bean and Banana Relish

This relish is rich with Cuban flavors, both sweet and intense. Serve this relish with any medium-bodied baked, steamed, or poached fish. It is just as good with a hot fish as with a chilled one. The relish is very low in calories and has almost no fat or sodium, while the red pepper and citrus juices are good sources of vitamin C. If you don't have any Black Beans with Orange and Jalapeño (page 108) on hand, any well-spiced black bean will do. This relish is best when served the same day it is prepared, and that is easy to do since the preparation takes only minutes. It also makes a delicious dip for toasted corn tortillas.

3/4 **banana, ripe but not soft**
1 **tablespoon fresh lime juice**
1 **tablespoon sweet red pepper**
1 **tablespoon green onion, sliced paper thin**
1/2 **cup Black Beans with Orange and Jalapeño, well rinsed of all starch (page 108)**
1/4 **cup freshly squeezed orange juice**
1 **teaspoon fresh cilantro, chopped fine**

The banana should be fully yellow and not yet turning soft. Carefully slice it lengthwise and then create uniformly shaped cubes no more than 1/4-inch wide. Carefully place the banana in the serving bowl and drizzle with the lime juice, to keep it from turning brown. Handle the banana as little as possible.

Keeping the ingredients separate in the serving bowl, create a very fine dice with the red pepper, about 1/8-inch thin. Do not use the white pulp in the relish, though you may want to eat it since it is high in soluble fiber and bioflavonoids.

Slice the onion as thinly and uniformly as possible with a very sharp, nonserrated knife. When you rinse the black beans, try to wash away any brown starchy substance, leaving round and intact beans.

Squeeze the orange juice and pour it over all of the ingredients in the bowl. Sprinkle the cilantro over the top and carefully fold the relish together with just a few motions.

Let the relish rest for about an hour in the refrigerator and serve.

SERVES 6

	Fat (g)	Cholesterol (g)	Sodium (mg)	Calories
Total Recipe	3.3	0	4.2	300
Per Portion	.3	0	.7	50

Fresh Tomato Salsa

This is a low-sodium and, of course, low-calorie way to spice up favorite Mexican treats. It is also rich in monounsaturated oil from the cilantro pesto that flavors it. If you wish to reduce your fat content on this one substantially, use 2 tablespoons of chopped fresh cilantro instead of pesto. This salsa is also very nice on fish. Look for vine-ripened tomatoes, or buy the red plum tomatoes sold year around and let them ripen further at room temperature.

3/4 cup fresh mild chili peppers, seeded and diced fine (cubanel or other mild peppers)

1½ teaspoons finely diced jalapeno pepper (about 1 medium pepper)

1½ cups finely diced fresh tomatoes (about 2–3 medium tomatoes)

1 tablespoon lemon juice

1 tablespoon Cilantro Pesto (page 94)

½ teaspoon black pepper, coarse grind

1¼ teaspoons chopped garlic

To prepare the jalapeño and mild chili peppers, wash and remove the stems. Slice the peppers lengthwise, and remove the seeds under cool running water. Mince the peppers, and immediately wash your hands with soap and warm water.

In a medium bowl, stir all the ingredients together, except the garlic.

In a food processor fitted with a metal blade, purée 1/3 of the tomato mixture with the garlic and stir back into the relish.

Let the relish rest at room temperature for at least 30 minutes, allowing the flavors to blend.

SERVES 6

	Fat (g)	Cholesterol (g)	Sodium (mg)	Calories
Total Recipe	72	0	276	840
Per Portion	12	0	46	140

Tomatilla Salsa

This relish is fat-free and is very low in sodium and calories. It can be used with many Mexican or Southwestern dishes, alone or with Fresh Tomato Salsa (page 168). Try it with Mexican Salad (page 124) or with Curried Black Beans (page 109). When serving the salsa as an accompaniment, use Thickest Yogurt (page 88) instead of sour cream. Tomatillas are Mexican and akin to a green tomato, without a lot of bitterness. They are available in most large supermarkets.

1 cup chopped tomatillas, outer skin and stem removed, cut into 1/4-inch pieces (6–8 medium tomatillas)
1/2 teaspoon minced fresh garlic, or to taste
2 teaspoons minced fresh jalapeño pepper, seeds removed
1/4 teaspoon grated fresh ginger root
1 tablespoon fresh lemon juice

In a food processor fitted with a metal blade, purée 1/2 cup of the tomatillas with the remaining ingredients. Taste the mixture and add a little extra garlic if you wish, keeping in mind that the garlic will increase in intensity over time.

Fold the remaining tomatillas into the purée.

Let the mixture rest for at least one hour before serving, so the flavors can blend.

SERVES 8
1 tablespoon per serving

	Fat (g)	Cholesterol (g)	Sodium (mg)	Calories
Total Recipe	0	0	43.8	138
Per Portion	0	0	5.5	17.3

Herbed Garlic Dressing

This is a very versatile dressing. It has all the flavor of an herbed mayonnaise or cheese without the fat. Use it as a dip for vegetables, brush it over hot vegetables, spread it on toasted bread like a cheese, or use it as a dressing on sandwiches. If you have access to fresh herbs, use them; otherwise, the dried variety will do. This dressing freezes well, so you can make a double batch and freeze half. Defrost it in the refrigerator overnight, and blend well before serving.

8 ounces soft tofu
¼ teaspoon dried leaf thyme (or 1 teaspoon fresh thyme)
½ teaspoon dried dill (or 1 tablespoon fresh dill)
½ teaspoon dried sweet basil (or 1 tablespoon fresh basil)
1 teaspoon dried parsley (or 1 tablespoon fresh parsley)
¼ teaspoon dried tarragon (or 1½ teaspoon fresh
** tarragon)**
1½ teaspoons chopped fresh garlic
½ teaspoon freshly ground black pepper
⅛ teaspoon cayenne pepper
1 tablespoon reduced-calorie mayonnaise
2 tablespoons nonfat plain yogurt
1 tablespoon fresh lemon juice

In a food processor fitted with a metal blade, purée the tofu, herbs, and garlic until creamy and light.

Add the remaining ingredients and blend.

Let the dressing rest in the refrigerator for at least an hour and adjust any of the herbs or spices to suit your taste.

Before serving, whip the sauce with a spoon until light. Makes about 1 cup.

SERVES 12
1 tablespoon per serving

	Fat (g)	Cholesterol (g)	Sodium (mg)	Calories
Total Recipe	8.4	0	254.4	240
Per Portion	.7	0	21.2	20

– Lemon Tarragon Dressing –

This sauce is virtually fat-free and low in sodium, and has the appearance of a mayonnaise-based dressing. It is delicious on cold or hot vegetables such as asparagus and broccoli or on sandwiches as a dressing. (See Focaccia sandwich with Asparagus and Lemon Tarragon Sauce, page 235.) If you'd like to lighten the texture of the sauce and give it a mild tartness, try replacing half of the tofu with plain nonfat yogurt. This freezes well, so you can make a double batch and freeze half. Defrost in the refrigerator overnight and blend well to serve.

4 ounces soft tofu
1 teaspoon grated lemon zest (yellow only, no white pulp)
1 teaspoon chopped shallot
2 tablespoons nonfat plain yogurt
1 tablespoon reduced-calorie mayonnaise
1 teaspoon dried tarragon (or 1 tablespoon fresh chopped
    tarragon)
1/16 teaspoon cayenne pepper (about 1 pinch)
1 tablespoon fresh lemon juice

In a food processor fitted with a metal blade, purée the tofu, lemon zest, and shallots until smooth and creamy.

Add the remaining ingredients and process until smooth and creamy.

Let the sauce chill in the refrigerator and adjust the pepper and tarragon to suit your taste.

Stir the sauce briskly before serving.

SERVES 6

	Fat (g)	Cholesterol (g)	Sodium (mg)	Calories
Total Recipe	4.8	.6	106.8	71.4
Per Portion	.8	.1	17.8	11.9

– Apricot and Sage Dressing –

This dressing is light and delicate and uses no oil. It also has the added beta-carotene of cooked carrots. Like Carrot and Tarragon Dressing (page 172), this dressing is mild and is best served with a tender lettuce such as butter or Boston lettuce or a chilled mild fish.

2/3 cup apricot nectar (a 5½-ounce can)
1 tablespoon soft-cooked carrot
1 teaspoon Ariél brand dealcoholized premium white wine
3 fresh sage leaves (or 1/4 teaspoon dried sage leaves)

Purée the apricot nectar and the cooked carrot. There should be no visible pieces of carrot.

Add the wine and sage leaves. Mince the sage beforehand if you are not using a food processor or blender.

SERVES 8

	Fat (g)	Cholesterol (g)	Sodium (mg)	Calories
Total Recipe	0	0	16	124
Per Portion	0	0	2	15.5

Carrot and Tarragon Dressing

This dressing is high in beta-carotene and essentially nonfat. Because it is very low in acid, it makes a mild dressing and should be used on delicately flavored lettuce or fish. Try it on butter or Boston lettuce or as a sauce served under cold poached flounder.

1/4 cup chopped peach (or pear), ripe and juicy
1/4 soft cooked carrot
1/2 cup pure carrot juice, unsweetened and unsalted
2 tablespoons Ariél brand dealcoholized premium white wine
1 tablespoon rice vinegar
1/2 teaspoon dried tarragon, or to taste (or 11/2 teaspoons fresh chopped tarragon)

In a food processor fitted with a metal blade, purée the ripe peach with the carrot and carrot juice.

Blend in the wine and rice vinegar. Add the tarragon and let it rest for an hour.

Taste the dressing and add more tarragon if it is too faint to detect. Be careful not to overpower the carrot flavor.

SERVES 10

	Fat (g)	Cholesterol (g)	Sodium (mg)	Calories
Total Recipe	1	0	65	176
Per Portion	.1	0	6.5	17.6

Papaya Coconut Dressing

This salad dressing is slightly sweet and fruity, is low in sodium and fat, and goes a long way. It is delicious served with Asian or Southwestern dishes. Try it tossed with peppery salad greens like arugula, endive, or mustard greens. Its flavor does something magical when drizzled over hot steamed spinach. Or, serve this dressing tossed with lettuce or drizzled over cold vegetables and fruit with a sprinkle of fresh cilantro. Use this sauce right away because the flavors tend to change after a day or so.

1/2 cup chopped fresh ripe papaya
5 teaspoons fresh lemon or lime juice
1 tablespoon rice vinegar
scant 1/4 teaspoon coconut extract
2 teaspoons sugar
1/4 teaspoon minced fresh ginger root
1 tablespoon safflower, corn, or canola oil
1/16 teaspoon cayenne pepper (about 1 large pinch), or to
    taste
1/8 teaspoon ground mace (about 2 large pinches)
chopped fresh cilantro, optional

In a food processor or blender fitted with a metal blade, blend the papaya, lemon juice, vinegar, coconut extract, sugar, and ginger root until smooth.

Very slowly drizzle in the oil, allowing it to emulsify. Add the pepper and mace.

SERVES 6

	Fat (g)	Cholesterol (g)	Sodium (mg)	Calories
Total Recipe	29.5	0	60	338
Per Portion	4.9	0	10	56.3

Pear Vinaigrette

This vinaigrette is naturally sweet and low in sodium. Surprisingly, the black pepper brings out the delicate pear flavor. Serve this vinaigrette on any tossed salad or with sliced vine-ripened tomatoes. It is also great as a dip for assorted cold fruits and vegetables.

2/3 cup ripe bosc pear, chopped (1 pear)
1/4 cup rice vinegar
1/2 cup extra virgin olive oil
2 teaspoons maple syrup
1/2 teaspoon cracked black pepper

In a food processor fitted with a metal blade, purée the pear with the vinegar until smooth.

Drizzle in the oil slowly so that it emulsifies. Add the maple syrup and pepper and blend.

SERVES 12 (approximately 1 tablespoon per serving)

	Fat (g)	Cholesterol (g)	Sodium (mg)	Calories
Total Recipe	82	0	1.1	817
Per Portion	7	0	.1	68

— Tomato Dill Vinaigrette —

This vinaigrette is low in acid and requires no salt to balance its flavor. Serve it with cold vegetables rather than on salads, because it is thicker than a salad dressing. For a variation, omit the dill and yogurt and serve over vegetables with a garnish of sliced fresh basil.

2 ripe plum tomatoes, or equivalent in vine-ripened variety
1 tablespoon chopped shallots
2 tablespoons extra virgin olive oil
1/2 teaspoon coarse black pepper
1 teaspoon dried dill (or 1 1/2 tablespoons chopped fresh
dill)
2 tablespoons nonfat plain yogurt

With a sharp paring knife, remove as much skin from the tomatoes as possible by simply peeling away from the stem base.

In a food processor fitted with metal blade, purée the tomatoes and shallots until smooth.

Drizzle the olive oil into the food processor, allowing it to blend with the tomato mixture. Add the pepper, dill, and yogurt.

SERVES 6

	Fat (g)	Cholesterol (g)	Sodium (mg)	Calories
Total Recipe	27	0	42	294
Per Portion	4.5	0	7	49

—— Shallot Vinaigrette ——

Shallot vinaigrette traditionally contains a lot of salt. This one is made with cooked carrot which adds a little sweetness, reducing the need for sodium. The carrot also adds beta-carotene and a nice color. This vinaigrette is low in fat and sodium and is robust. Serve it with heartier lettuces like romaine or arugula. It is also delicious as a marinade for steamed, chilled vegetables.

1 tablespoon red wine vinegar
1/2 teaspoon freshly ground black pepper
1 tablespoon soft-cooked carrot
1 tablespoon plus 1 teaspoon extra virgin olive oil
2 tablespoons Low-Sodium Chicken Stock (see page 88)
1 teaspoon sugar

In a food processor fitted with a metal blade, purée the vinegar, pepper, and carrot until smooth.

Drizzle in oil in a stream, allowing it to emulsify.

Add chicken stock and sugar.

SERVES 6

	Fat (g)	Cholesterol (g)	Sodium (mg)	Calories
Total Recipe	13.2	0	76.2	219.6
Per Portion	2.2	0	12.7	36.6

Caesar Dressing

Caesar dressing is usually off limits for those avoiding sodium and fat. This one is full of flavor but low in fat and sodium, because it uses sardines instead of anchovies. If you like a mild anchovy flavor, use 1 sardine instead of 2. Toss this dressing with crisp romaine lettuce. Keep this dressing well chilled until ready to use. Use it right away, because of the egg white.

1–2 sardines, canned in water, no salt or fat added
3 tablespoons fresh lemon juice
1 teaspoon fresh garlic, minced
2 tablespoons freshly grated Parmesan cheese
1 tablespoon extra virgin olive oil
1 egg white, well chilled

In a food processor fitted with a metal blade, purée the sardines, lemon juice, and garlic. Add the olive oil in a slow stream.

Make sure your egg has been well chilled. Add the egg white and allow the dressing to blend for a moment.

Finally, add the freshly grated Parmesan cheese.

SERVES 8

	Fat (g)	Cholesterol (g)	Sodium (mg)	Calories
Total Recipe	20	11.2	311.2	253.6
Per Portion	2.5	1.4	38.9	31.7

—— Poached Salmon Fillet ——

This is a simple way to poach fish while retaining its moisture and flavor. Use the method with any fish. The stock and wine impart taste while preserving the delicate moisture, leaving little need for fatty sauces. Try yogurt or tofu-based sauces, or one of the relishes. Salmon is very high in Omega-3 fatty acids.

> **1¼ pounds salmon, filleted and skinned**
> **1 cup Ariél brand dealcoholized premium dry white wine**
> **2 cups Low-Sodium Chicken Stock (page 88) or Vegetable**
>   **Stock (page 90)**
> **3 large sprigs of fresh dill (other herbs may be used)**
> **water to cover if necessary**

Trim any fatty pieces from the edges of the salmon. Place the fish in a baking dish just larger than the fish and cover with the dill. Preheat the oven to 375° F.

Pour in the wine and cover the fish with stock. Cover the dish.

Place in a hot oven and let it cook for about 15 minutes. The center should be almost fully cooked, or approaching opaqueness like the edges. It will continue to cook outside the oven.

Remove the pan. If the center is not fully cooked, let the fish rest in the covered baking dish and it will continue to cook.

SERVES 4
4 ounces per serving

	Fat (g)	Cholesterol (g)	Sodium (mg)	Calories
Total Recipe	51	336	402	1302
Per Portion	8.5	56	67	217

— Salmon with Potato Crust —

This makes an interesting presentation at the table. It is low in fat and sodium and high in Omega-3 fatty acids. Serve it with fresh lemon.

1 pound salmon fillets, center cut and skinless
1½ cups shredded or matchstick-cut potatoes
1 egg white, lightly beaten
2 teaspoons safflower, sunflower, corn, or canola oil
1 tablespoon fresh lemon juice

Cut the salmon at an angle and against the grain into four equal-sized pieces. The thinner the salmon, the better.

Whip the egg white until frothy. Dry the fillets with white paper towels and brush with the egg white.

With the potato pieces in your hands, lightly press them onto the fish wedge as if making a patty. Cover the fillets with the potato pieces as much as possible and pat them into place, forming an encasement. Refrigerate the potato-covered fish, uncovered, about 20 minutes, to dry the egg white. Preheat the oven to 350° F.

Heat the oil in a heavy skillet, either seasoned or nonstick, over medium-high heat. When the pan is hot, carefully place two pieces of fish in the pan, bottom side down. Let the potato crisp on medium-high heat about three minutes. Turn the fillet over when the potato has turned golden brown. Let the top side crisp and remove the fish to a baking sheet. Let the pan heat again, and repeat the process with the remaining 2 pieces.

Roast the fish on the baking sheet in a 350° F oven for about 10 minutes, or until the center is nearly opaque. The fish will continue to cook as it rests.

Drizzle with lemon juice just before serving.

SERVES 4
4 ounces per serving

	Fat (g)	Cholesterol (g)	Sodium (mg)	Calories
Total Recipe	40	210	312	988
Per Portion	10	52.3	78	247

Garlic-Laced Shad

Shad is so tender and subtle that it cries out for a simple preparation such as this. Shad is lower in cholesterol than many fish. Make sure the shad is fresh and is free of all bones; a professional must fillet the fish, since it has a very complex structure of fine bones.

1 pound boned shad, skin on
1 teaspoon olive oil
1 teaspoon minced fresh garlic
vegetable oil spray
1/2 teaspoon freshly ground black pepper
4 fresh lemon slices for garnish

Preheat the oven to 350°F. In a small bowl, blend the olive oil and garlic. Spray a baking dish with vegetable oil spray and lay the shad in the pan.

Gently spread the mixture on the top side of the shad. Bake the fish at 350° F for about 15 minutes, or until the thickest portion has changed from translucent to opaque and is still moist and tender.

As you remove the fish from the pan, leave the skin behind. Serve with fresh lemon slices.

SERVES 4

	Fat (g)	Cholesterol (g)	Sodium (mg)	Calories
Total Recipe	49.6	trace	245	815.6
Per Portion	12.4	trace	61.25	203.9

Rainbow Trout
Stewed with Tomato

This fish stew has a Tuscan zest, all the benefits of fresh fish, and less fat than most sauces. It can be served alone, with crusty bread like Focaccia with Fresh Sage (page 224), or over pasta. Try to use the ripest fresh tomatoes you can. In the winter months most supermarkets carry plum tomatoes, which can be further ripened at home at room temperature for a day or so.

1 pound skinless rainbow trout fillets or other flavorful fish
1¼ cups sliced leek, dark green portion removed (about 1 leek)
1 teaspoon extra virgin olive oil
1¼ cups thinly sliced onion (about 1 large onion)
2 stalks of celery, leaves removed and sliced in ⅛-inch pieces
¾ teaspoon dried thyme
¾ teaspoon dried rosemary
½ teaspoon red pepper flakes
½ bay leaf
1 cup Ariél brand dealcoholized premium dry white wine
3 fresh plum tomatoes, or 2 medium-ripe tomatoes, cut in sixths
2 tablespoons chopped fresh parsley
1½ cups Low-Sodium Chicken Stock (page 88)
4 teaspoons freshly grated Parmesan cheese

Split the leek several times up the center, keeping the roots intact. Rinse the leek thoroughly under cold running water, making sure all sand and debris are gone. Cut off the darkest green portion and slice the remainder in ⅓-inch pieces.

Heat the olive oil in a heavy, nonaluminum skillet over medium-high heat. Sauté the onion for about 5 minutes or until the edges become translucent. Add the leeks, celery, herbs, and spices. Stir briefly and sauté until the herbs release their aroma.

Add the wine and simmer for about 5 minutes, reducing by half.

Meanwhile, slice each fish fillet on an angle, creating 2- to 3-inch wide pieces. Try to create a total of 12 pieces.

Add the tomato, parsley, and stock to the pan and stir. Immerse the fish in the stock and cook over low heat about 10 minutes, until the edges start to curl.

Remove the fish to a covered plate and reduce the stock by half, about 10 minutes. The celery should be tender. Remove and discard the bay leaf.

Serve in shallow bowls with Parmesan cheese sprinkled on top.

SERVES 4

	Fat (g)	Cholesterol (g)	Sodium (mg)	Calories
Total Recipe	32.8	381.6	2544	1520
Per Portion	8.2	95.4	636	380

— Tuna Fillet with Wasabi, — Ginger, and Sweet Red Pepper

Both the tuna and its preparation are naturally low in calories, fat, cholesterol, and sodium. The wasabi (horseradish) and ginger are surprisingly refreshing and mildly spicy with the tuna. The wasabi is available in the gourmet section of the supermarket or in Asian markets.

1 pound tuna steaks (4 steaks)
4 teaspoons wasabi powder
4 teaspoons water
4 teaspoons rice vinegar
2 teaspoons grated fresh ginger root
1 sweet red pepper, cut into 1/8-inch sticks
1/2 teaspoon cracked black pepper

In a very small bowl, mix the wasabi powder with the water until smooth. Then stir in the vinegar and ginger.

Broil the steaks for 2–3 minutes on the first side.

Turn the steaks over, coat with the wasabi mixture, and sprinkle with the pepper. Broil for an additional 2–3 minutes close to the element until done. Try to let the edges brown slightly without cooking the meat too long.

Meanwhile, heat a large, nonstick skillet or wok over medium-high heat, and stir-fry the peppers until softened but still firm. If a nonstick pan is not available, use vegetable oil spray.

Serve the steaks with pepper sticks gracing their edges like pick-up sticks.

SERVES 4
1 steak per serving

	Fat (g)	Cholesterol (g)	Sodium (mg)	Calories
Total Recipe	26.8	210	217.6	808
Per Portion	6.7	52.5	54.4	202

Tuna with Avocado Papaya Relish

Tuna is naturally low in sodium, fat, and calories, and this relish enjoys the vitamin C and beta-carotene benefits of papaya and sweet red pepper without extra sodium or fat. If you can, use fresh herbs; it makes all the difference with this relish. Serve the relish with just about any medium-bodied fish, or as a dip with firm lettuce leaves like radicchio or romaine. Try serving Gingered Rolls (page 225) with this meal. If you don't have Cilantro Pesto on hand, this recipe is enjoyable without it.

4 4-ounce tuna steaks, center cut
1 tablespoon Cilantro Pesto (page 94)
1/2 California avocado, ripe and firm, cut into 1/4-inch cubes
1/2 cup papaya, peeled, seeds removed, and cut into 1/4-inch cubes
1 jalapeño pepper, seeds removed, minced
1 tablespoon minced red onion
2 tablespoons red pepper, without any white pulp, cut into 1/4-inch cubes
1/4 teaspoon minced fresh garlic
1/2 teaspoon cracked black pepper
3 tablespoons fresh lemon juice
1 tablespoon rice vinegar
1 tablespoon fresh cilantro, chopped (or 1 tablespoon chopped fresh parsley and 1/4 teaspoon dried cilantro)
1 tablespoon fresh basil, chopped (or 1/2 teaspoon dried sweet basil)

Place the ingredients in a shallow serving bowl as they are cut. After cutting the avocado, sprinkle the pieces with 1 tablespoon of the lemon juice, to keep them from turning brown. Handle the ingredients as little as possible and keep them separate at this point. There should be equal portions of papaya and avocado.

With all of the ingredients in the serving bowl except the basil and cilantro, sprinkle the remaining lemon juice and the rice vinegar over the top. Using a large rubber spatula, fold the mixture together gently in a few strokes, being careful not to bruise or smear the cubes of fruit. Let the relish rest in the refrigerator for about an hour. Remove it to room temperature while you prepare the tuna.

While the relish is resting, rub the tuna steaks with the Cilantro Pesto and broil them for 1–2 minutes on each side. The center should be mostly opaque.

Just before serving, fold the cilantro and basil into the relish.

Serve the tuna with the relish gracing one side.

SERVES 4

	Fat (g)	Cholesterol (g)	Sodium (mg)	Calories
Total Recipe	31.8	204	235.6	866
Per Portion	7.95	51	58.9	216.5

Grouper with Sweet Peppers and Potatoes

This fish is laced with the sweetness of red peppers, sweet potatoes, and fresh marjoram. The sweet potatoes provide beta-carotene and the peppers provide vitamin C. The sauce is low in fat, and the grouper is high in Omega-3 fatty acids.

1/2 pound sweet potato
1 pound grouper fillet
1/2 cup peeled and chopped shallots (2–3 medium shallots)
1 large sweet red pepper, halved and sliced 1/8 inch thick
1/2 cup Ariél brand dealcoholized premium dry white wine
1 cup Low-Sodium Chicken Stock (page 88)
2 teaspoons fresh marjoram, chopped (or 3/4 teaspoon dried marjoram)
1 teaspoon extra virgin olive oil
1/16 teaspoon cayenne pepper (about 1 large pinch)
1 tablespoon freshly grated Parmesan cheese

Preheat the oven to 375° F. Bake the potatoes for about 35 minutes or until a sharp knife slides out easily. They should be cooked but still firm.

Peel and slice the potatoes into 1/4-inch slices and set aside. (If the potatoes are large, halve them before slicing.) Reduce the oven to 350° F.

Heat the olive oil over medium-high heat in a medium-to-large heavy skillet and add the shallots.

Sauté the shallots for about a minute or until they start to turn translucent. Add the sweet pepper and cook for 2 minutes longer or until it starts to soften.

Add the wine and simmer until only a syrup is left. Add the stock and potatoes and simmer for 1 minute. Toss with the marjoram and set aside.

Meanwhile, lay the grouper in an ungreased baking dish and bake in a 350° F oven for 10–15 minutes, or until the center is almost opaque. Allow about 10 minutes per inch of thickness at the thickest point. Remove the fish, cover with the completed sauce, and surround with the potato pieces before returning to the oven for 5 minutes more.

Remove the fish to a platter, surround the fish with the potato slices, cover with the sauce, and lace the top with Parmesan cheese.

SERVES 4

	Fat (g)	Cholesterol (g)	Sodium (mg)	Calories
Total Recipe	12.8	175.2	457.2	809.6
Per Portion	3.2	43.8	114.3	202.4

—— Warmed Oysters with —— Spinach and Papaya

Oysters are low in sodium, calories, and fat, and this recipe has the added nutrition of spinach and papaya for beta-carotene. Serve the dressing cold with the warmed oysters. Try warmed oysters with Black Bean and Banana Relish (page 166) or with Papaya and Citrus Relish (page 165).

24 raw fresh oysters, shucked and on the half shell
2 cups raw spinach
1/2 recipe Papaya Coconut Dressing (page 172)
1 teaspoon black sesame seeds

Preheat the oven to 400°F. After thoroughly soaking and washing the spinach, remove the tough stems and steam it until it is just wilted.

Place the shucked oysters, in their shells, in a baking pan. Divide the spinach among the oysters, layering several leaves on each shell. Bake the oysters for 3–4 minutes, or until they have lost their translucence and are slightly puffed.

Spoon 1–2 teaspoons of the dressing on each oyster. Top with sesame seeds and serve immediately.

SERVES 4
6 oysters per serving

	Fat (g)	Cholesterol (g)	Sodium (mg)	Calories
Total Recipe	8.8	184	464	248
Per Portion	2.2	46	116	62

Yellowtail Sole with Sesame Seeds and Black Pepper

This is a simple and amazingly subtle preparation that can be used for any mild fish. Serve this fish alone or with one of the relishes in this book, like Tuna with Avocado Papaya Relish (page 182), or Papaya and Citrus Relish (page 165).

vegetable oil spray
2 tablespoons sesame seeds
1 teaspoon cracked black pepper
4 sole fillets, about 1 pound

Preheat oven to 350° F. To pan-roast the sesame seeds, spray a small sauté or frying pan with vegetable oil spray and cook them over medium-high heat until their aroma is released and they start to turn golden. Watch them carefully so they don't burn.

Mix the sesame seeds with the pepper.

Gently press the seed mixture onto the fillets and bake at 350° F for about 5 minutes, or until the center just turns opaque. This fish is extremely tender, so don't overdo it.

SERVES 4

	Fat (g)	Cholesterol (g)	Sodium (mg)	Calories
Total Recipe	14	216	375	511
Per Portion	3.5	54	93.75	127.75

Sole and Pecan Rolls

This is a very mild fish and the pecans add a subtle flavor. This preparation can be used for any mild flat fish. Serve it with colorful vegetables, since its color is on the pale side. Try serving it with Gingered Carrots (page 151) and steamed spinach with Papaya Coconut Dressing (page 172). If you like, use cashews or walnuts instead of pecans.

12 sole fillets, about 1 pound
¼ cup chopped pecans
vegetable oil spray

Preheat the oven to 350° F and roast the pecans on a baking sheet for about 10 minutes, turning after 5 minutes. The pecans should just start to brown and release their aroma.

Gently roll up the fillets, and touch the outer side to the chopped nuts, picking up as many nuts as possible.

Place them seam side down on a baking sheet sprayed with vegetable oil spray.

Bake in a 350° F oven for about 15 minutes.

SERVES 4

	Fat (g)	Cholesterol (g)	Sodium (mg)	Calories
Total Recipe	25.2	216	368	610.4
Per Portion	6.3	54	92	152.6

— Poached Chicken Breasts —

If you need white chicken meat for lunch salads or sandwiches and you don't have the time to make a chicken stock, you can poach individual chicken breasts. Serve them hot or cold, sliced on salads or sandwiches, or as a main course with any number of relishes and sauces. (See the section on sauces, page 154.) Poached chicken breasts can be as tender as butter, but are extremely low in fat and calories, and fairly low in sodium.

 4 chicken breast halves, about 1 pound
 2 cups Low-Sodium Chicken Stock (page 88), or water
 1 bay leaf
 1 teaspoon dried thyme
 1/2 teaspoon black peppercorns

Place the chicken in a heavy, medium saucepan, layering it if necessary. Cover the chicken with the herbs and stock.

Bring the pot to a simmer and reduce the heat to low. Cook for about 10 minutes or until the chicken is cooked but still soft and tender. Do not boil. The lower the temperature, the more tender the chicken will be.

Remove the chicken to stop the cooking. Bring the stock to a boil, strain, and refrigerate (or freeze) for future use.

SERVES 4

	Fat (g)	Cholesterol (g)	Sodium (mg)	Calories
Total Recipe	12.4	292	252	568
Per Portion	3.1	73	63	142

—— Crispy Roasted Chicken ——

This chicken has its own special appeal compared to fatty fried chicken or the very salty commercial chicken coatings. If you must use prepared bread crumbs, add approximately 120 milligrams of sodium to each serving. Try substituting your favorite herbs or use your favorite poultry instead of chicken.

1 teaspoon chopped garlic
3/4 cup low-sodium bread crumbs, made from Crusty Italian
    Bread (page 223) or other low-sodium bread
1/4 teaspoon dried thyme
1/2 teaspoon dried rosemary
1/2 teaspoon black pepper
4 chicken breast halves

To prepare the bread crumbs, let about 1 1/2 slices of bread dry out; a low setting on a toaster oven will help. When the bread is dry enough to crumble, grind it in a blender until fine, or enclose it in a linen towel and roll with a rolling pin. Remove the crumbs and measure.

Mix the garlic, bread crumbs, thyme, rosemary, and pepper in a blender until they are fine and blended. Preheat the oven to 375° F.

Remove all visible fat and skin from the chicken. Toss the chicken in the herbed bread crumbs. (Do not save the crumb mixture as it has been exposed to the raw chicken.)

Roast the chicken on a baking sheet about 25–30 minutes, or until the center is opaque and very light pink, depending on the size of the breasts. The meat will continue to cook outside the oven.

SERVES 4

	Fat (g)	Cholesterol (g)	Sodium (mg)	Calories
Total Recipe	16	292	258	872
Per Portion	4	73	64.5	208

Southwestern Chicken

This is a simple combination of Cilantro Pesto and the very low-fat chicken breast. The secret to this dish is to avoid cooking it at a high heat and remove it from the heat when the center is no longer translucent but shows a hint of pink; it will continue cooking and produce a very tender piece of meat. Serve it with Fresh Tomato Salsa or sliced thin for a sandwich or salad.

1 pound chicken breasts (4 pieces)
1 tablespoon Cilantro Pesto (page 94)
2 tablespoons unsalted pepitas (pumpkin seeds)

Preheat the oven to 350°F and roast the pepitas on a nonstick baking sheet for 5–7 minutes. Keep watch so they don't burn. Trim the chicken of all visible fat and skin and spread the pesto on the top side.

Turn the oven to 375° F. Rough chop the pepitas and tamp them lightly into the pesto.

Put a very small amount of water in the bottom of the roasting pan (just enough to cover the bottom) and place the chicken in the pan, pesto side up. Roast the chicken in a 375° F oven for about 20 minutes. (The water will evaporate eventually but will help the meat stay moist.) The center can be very light pink when you remove them, because they will continue to cook as they rest. Remove them to a covered dish.

SERVES 4

	Fat (g)	Cholesterol (g)	Sodium (mg)	Calories
Total Recipe	30	292	458	821.2
Per Portion	7.5	73	114.5	205.3

Turkey with Oregano and Mushrooms

Turkey breast is low in fat, sodium, and calories. This recipe indulges with a little cheese and the end product seems more sinful than it actually is.

4 turkey breast cutlets
1/2 teaspoon freshly ground black pepper
1/8 teaspoon cayenne pepper, about 2 large pinches
1/2 pound fresh mushrooms, sliced 1/4-inch thick
1/2 cup Ariél brand dealcoholized premium dry white wine
1 1/2 teaspoons fresh oregano, chopped, or 1/4 teaspoon
      dried leaf oregano
4 ounces low-sodium swiss cheese, sliced
vegetable oil spray

Heat a large, heavy, nonstick skillet over medium-high heat. While the pan is heating up, dry the cutlets with a white paper towel and sprinkle with the peppers. Spray the pan with vegetable oil spray.

Sauté two cutlets at a time for about 1 minute on each side. Remove them to a baking dish. Let the pan get hot again before finishing the last two.

In the hot pan, sauté the mushrooms, cooking for 2–3 minutes or until they are lightly browned and tender but have not started to shrink and give off liquid. Remove them to a bowl.

Add the wine to the pan. Reduce it by half its volume, stirring up any meat and mushroom juices. Remove wine to the mushroom bowl.

Sprinkle the cutlets with oregano and top with the cheese. Broil close to the heat source for about 2 minutes, or until the cheese starts to bubble, but not brown.

Top with the mushrooms and their juices.

SERVES 4

	Fat (g)	Cholesterol (g)	Sodium (mg)	Calories
Total Recipe	39.6	314.8	360.4	956
Per Portion	9.9	78.7	90.1	239

Special Hamburgers

These hamburgers use a leaner cut of beef and have added ingredients to perk up a traditional treat without a lot of salty condiments. Try making your own low-sodium Ketchup (page 154) or serve with Barbecue Sauce (page 154). You might serve these hamburgers with Peppered Yam Fries (page 136).

1 pound ground round of beef
2 tablespoons minced onion
4 tablespoons minced sweet red pepper
2 tablespoons chopped fresh parsley
4 teaspoons Worcestershire sauce
2 teaspoons no-salt-added Dijon mustard
1/8 teaspoon cayenne pepper (about 2 large pinches), or to taste
1/4 teaspoon garlic powder, or to taste

Combine the ingredients well and form 4 patties.

Heat a heavy, nonstick skillet over medium-high heat. Dust the patties with garlic powder and saute for 3–5 minutes on each side.

Serve with Barbecue Sauce (page 154) or Ketchup (page 154) alone or in a sandwich. Or, as an alternative, spread a small amount of Herbed Garlic Dressing (page 169) over the top, or serve with Horseradish Sauce (page 160).

SERVES 4
1 hamburger per serving

	Fat (g)	Cholesterol (g)	Sodium (mg)	Calories
Total Recipe	32	340	571.6	1200
Per Portion	8	85	142.9	300

Flank Steak

Flank steak is one of the most flavorful of the cuts of beef and is also very low in fat. When well prepared, it can become the backdrop for many lovely sauces. Try serving it with Horseradish Sauce (page 160) or Roasted Red Pepper Relish (page 163) For a variation, try rubbing the meat with 1 teaspoon of your favorite herb combination such as rosemary and black pepper.

1 pound flank steak
1 clove garlic, minced

Trim all visible fat and "silver skin" from the meat.

Rub the steak with the garlic and let it sit in the refrigerator for about 15 minutes.

Broil the steak at close range to crisp the outside without overcooking the center. Broil the meat for 5 minutes on the first side and 3 minutes on the second side.

Always let the steak rest for about 5 minutes before cutting; otherwise the juices will be lost. Turn the first side up and slice very thinly.

SERVES 4

	Fat (g)	Cholesterol (g)	Sodium (mg)	Calories
Total Recipe	50.8	360	367.2	1248
Per Portion	12.7	60	61.2	208

Sesame-Marinated Beef

This marinated beef has all the flavor of teriyaki without the sodium added by soy sauce. It is rich in sesame flavor and low in fat. It is also fairly low in calories and cholesterol. Instead of serving it as a steak, you might try slicing it very thinly across the grain and stir-frying it in a hot skillet or wok. Or stir fry it with sliced green and red sweet peppers for a less salty version of Chinese pepper steak. It also makes a very nice meat for sandwiches or salads. Try serving it hot on a garden salad tossed with Papaya and Coconut Dressing (page 172).

1 pound top round steak, cut 1/4 inch thick
1 tablespoon freshly minced garlic
2 teaspoons sesame oil
1 teaspoon black pepper
2 tablespoons fresh lime juice (juice of 2–3 limes)
1 tablespoon rice vinegar

Trim the steak of all visible fat and cut into 4 equal pieces.

In a nonaluminum pan or bowl, combine the garlic, sesame oil, pepper, lime juice, and rice vinegar. Submerge the steak pieces in the marinade and coat the meat thoroughly. Let it rest in the refrigerator for 1–1 1/2 hours, turning every half hour.

Heat a large, heavy nonstick skillet over medium-high heat. When the pan is hot, sauté 2 pieces of the meat at a time, 1–2 minutes on each side. Remove the meat, let the pan get hot again and repeat. The secret is to let the meat form a glazed crust from the marinade juices. This is done quickly in a hot pan so that the meat does not overcook or start to produce juices, which will lower the pan temperature.

Serve sliced thinly.

SERVES 4
3–4 ounces per serving

	Fat (g)	Cholesterol (g)	Sodium (mg)	Calories
Total Recipe	30.8	340	178.8	1064
Per Portion	7.7	85	44.7	266

— Spiced Pork Tenderloin —

This roast is as tender as and possibly more flavorful than popular beef tenderloin, with much less fat. The spices give it punch without adding much extra sodium. And it makes great leftovers for sandwiches.

1 pork tenderloin (approximately 3/4 pound)
1 teaspoon chili powder
1/2 teaspoon garlic powder
1/2 teaspoon dried oregano
1/2 teaspoon curry powder
1/8 teaspoon cayenne pepper (about 2 large pinches)
2 teaspoons hot pepper sauce, Louisiana-style, or Hot Sauce
   (page 155)

Preheat oven to 375° F. In a small bowl, combine the dry ingredients.
   Trim pork of all visible fat and "silver skin" and roll in the dry mixture.
   Roast the meat in a pre-heated 375° F oven for 25 minutes.
   Remove from oven to a cool platter and cover with the hot sauce.
   Let rest for 10 minutes and serve sliced very thinly. Drizzle with the hot sauce and meat drippings from the platter.
SERVES 4

	Fat (g)	Cholesterol (g)	Sodium (mg)	Calories
Total Recipe	42	300	347.2	868
Per Portion	10.5	75	86.8	207

— Roasted Pork Tenderloin with Fresh Thyme —

As a roast for a weekend traditional dinner, this one lacks the fat of beef roasts but has all the satisfaction. As simple as it is to prepare, the aromatics announce its arrival as it cooks.

1 pork tenderloin (approximately 3/4 pound)
1/2 teaspoon extra virgin olive oil
1/2 teaspoon minced fresh garlic
1 tablespoon fresh thyme leaves (or 1/2 teaspoon dried leaf
   thyme)

Preheat the oven to 375° F. Trim pork of all visible fat and "silver skin."

Heat a large, heavy, seasoned or nonstick skillet over medium-high heat. Coat the pork with olive oil and sear in the hot pan until golden brown on all sides.

Rub pork with minced garlic and coat with thyme leaves.

Roast in a pre-heated 375° F oven for 20 minutes.

Remove the roast and let it rest for 10 minutes. Serve sliced very thinly with its own meat juices.

SERVES 4

	Fat (g)	Cholesterol (g)	Sodium (mg)	Calories
Total Recipe	27.2	333.2	238	680
Per Portion	6.8	83.3	59.5	170

—— Pork Loin Chops with —— Lemon and Rosemary

This pork loin chop is fairly low in fat and sodium, and its crust adds flavor without the need for a rich, salty sauce. Although dried rosemary will do, try to use the fresh variety. It's well worth the effort on this one.

4 pork loin chops (about 5¹/₃ ounces each before cooking)
2 tablespoons fresh rosemary, chopped (or 1 tablespoon dried rosemary)
4 teaspoons grated fresh lemon zest
4 lemon wedges, optional

Remove all visible fat from the chops and pat dry with white paper towels. Preheat the oven to 350° F.

Heat a heavy skillet over medium-high-to-high heat. When the pan is hot, sear the chops to brown each side, no more than 1 minute on each side. Prepare 2 chops at a time and let the pan reheat before continuing.

Combine the rosemary and lemon zest and lightly press the mixture onto the chops, using the majority of the mixture for the top side.

Roast the chops in a nonaluminum baking pan for about 10 minutes or until light pink at the bone. Remove the chops to a plate to stop the cooking.

Serve with fresh lemon wedges if desired.

SERVES 4
3.5 ounces per serving

	Fat (g)	Cholesterol (g)	Sodium (mg)	Calories
Total Recipe	31.2	284	228	685.2
Per Portion	7.8	71	57	171.3

Pork Chops with Mustard Crust

Mustard is a great partner with pork and this one offers all the flavor and interest without the sodium. The pork is relatively low in fat compared to other pork choices. Try mixing a few pine nuts or walnuts with the bread crumbs; merely add 1.2 grams of fat and 12 calories per serving.

4 pork loin chops, about 6 ounces each with bone
4 teaspoons low-sodium Dijon mustard
2 tablespoons bread crumbs, unseasoned
1 tablespoon chopped pine nuts or walnuts, optional

Trim all fat from the chops.

Sear two chops at a time in a hot pan until they are brown, about 1 minute on each side. Use vegetable oil spray if the pan is not seasoned or nonstick.

Coat the top of each chop with half the mustard and lightly press the bread crumbs onto the mustard.

Broil the first side for about 3 minutes, turn and repeat the process for the second side.

SERVES 4

	Fat (g)	Cholesterol (g)	Sodium (mg)	Calories
Total Recipe	35.6	284	373.6	806
Per Portion	8.9	71	93.4	201.5

Pork Chops with Jalapeño Glaze

This simple recipe goes a long way when served with the right complements, like Southwestern Corn Bread (page 222) and Fresh Tomato Salsa (page 168). Or, try coating a trimmed pork tenderloin roast with the same ingredients.

4 pork loin chops (about 5^1/3 ounces each before cooking)
2 tablespoons jalapeño jelly
1 jalapeño pepper

Trim all visible fat from the chops.

Sear two chops at a time in a hot pan until they are brown, about 1 minute on each side. Use vegetable oil spray if the pan is not seasoned or non-stick.

Meanwhile, melt the jelly in a warm pan. Wash the jalapeño pepper with cold water and slice it in half lengthwise. Under cold running water remove the seeds with a small knife or your fingers, and slice into slivers. Be careful to wash your hands right away with soap and warm water, since the seeds leave a powerful resin.

Brush half the jelly onto the chops and broil for 2–3 minutes.

Brush the remainder of the jelly onto the chops and top with the jalapeño slices. Broil for 2–3 minutes longer until the meat at the bone is very light pink.

SERVES 4

	Fat (g)	Cholesterol (g)	Sodium (mg)	Calories
Total Recipe	30	284	236	884
Per Portion	7.5	71	59	221

Roasted Pork with Goat Cheese and Kale

This pork roast is packed with garlic and satisfying goat cheese flavor. Serve it with Roasted New Potatoes with Rosemary (page 136) or Peppered Yam Fries (page 136). Low-fat goat cheese is available in many gourmet markets; if you can't find it, try using Herbed Ricotta Cheese (page 233).

3 pounds rolled pork loin roast
1/4 pound fresh kale (or small leaves of collard greens)
2 ounces low-fat goat cheese or Herbed Ricotta Cheese (page 233)
1 clove fresh elephant garlic (or 2 large fresh garlic cloves)
1 teaspoon fresh, coarsely ground black pepper
1 teaspoon dried leaf thyme
kitchen twine

Preheat oven to 450° F. Wash and remove the stems from the kale.

Steam the greens (see page 87). Remove from the cooking pan and cool in the refrigerator. Pat dry.

Untie the roast if it has been rolled already and trim it of all visible fat. Make a 1/3-inch slit down the center of both halves of the roast. This will serve as a trough for the kale roll.

Lay the kale out in a rectangle the same width as the roast and 2 inches longer on each end lengthwise. With your hands, form the cheese into a tube the length of the roast and place it in the center of the kale. Fold the 2-inch ends over the cheese roll. Fold one of the long sides of kale neatly over the cheese, and roll the kale firmly around the goat cheese.

Place the kale roll in the center of the roast, resting on the trough. Replace the top of the roast and re-tie it carefully in at least four places. Do not cut off the extra kale that may hang out the ends of the roast, or the cheese will leak out.

Cut the elephant garlic clove in half and then slice each half paper thin, about 12 pieces total. With a very sharp paring knife, make 12 slits evenly around the roast and insert the garlic pieces.

Mix the thyme and pepper together and roll the roast in the mixture.

With the meat in a roasting pan, place the roast in the preheated 425° F oven. Close the door and reduce the heat to 325° F. Cook for 1–1 1/4 hours. Remove to a plate and let rest at least 15 minutes before slicing.

SERVES 12

	Fat (g)	Cholesterol (g)	Sodium (mg)	Calories
Total Recipe	159.4	1017	901	2860
Per Portion	13.3	84.7	75	238.3

— Rosemary-Marinated Leg — of Lamb

With such a flavorful preparation as this lower-fat cut of lamb, a little goes a long way. Try serving this robust meat in the summer with Green Beans Vinaigrette (page 116) and Focaccia with Fresh Sage (page 224) or Crusty Italian Bread (page 223). It is also delicious in colder months served with Spicy White Lima Beans (page 107).

¼ cup plus 1 tablespoon fresh rosemary leaves, chopped, or 2 tablespoons dried rosemary
2 tablespoons chopped garlic
1 teaspoon red pepper flakes
½ cup Ariél brand dealcoholized premium dry red wine
1 tablespoon red wine vinegar
1 tablespoon cracked black pepper
¼ cup extra virgin olive oil
2–2½ pounds leg of lamb, deboned and butterflied

Trim all visible fat and "silver skin" from the lamb and open it flat to a uniform thickness. If your butcher cannot butterfly it, simply slice into the thickest portions to open them out.

Whisk together the rosemary, garlic, wine, vinegar, oil, and peppers.

In a baking dish or bowl the size of the meat or in a plastic zip-lock bag, submerge the meat in the marinade. Make sure it is covered well with plastic wrap and refrigerate for 12–36 hours; the longer it marinates, the more flavor it develops.

When ready to prepare, cut the meat into two equal pieces. Preheat the oven to 375° F.

Heat a large, heavy sauté pan and sear both sides of the meat for 2–3 minutes on each side. This should form a crust on the meat. Prepare only one piece at a time, remove it to a baking dish, let the pan get hot again, and repeat for the second piece.

Roast the lamb for 20–25 minutes in a 375° F oven. If you like, you can roast the meat with the marinade in the bottom of the pan.

Remove the meat to a covered platter. While you're letting the meat rest for about 10 minutes, skim off all fat from the marinade and reduce in a small saucepan until only half its volume remains.

Slice the lamb very thinly across the grain, drizzle with the marinade and serve.

SERVES 10

	Fat (g)	Cholesterol (g)	Sodium (mg)	Calories
Total Recipe	118.4	560	782.4	2272
Per Portion	11.8	56	78.2	227.2

Roasted Veal

This is one of the least fatty and lowest calorie cuts of veal you can buy; veal flank is one of the most flavorful cuts. When prepared carefully, it can be extremely tender. Ask your butcher to save the flanks for you. You can also broil it (page 200). Serve it with Raspberry Sauce (page 162) or Wild Mushroom Sauce (page 161).

1½ pound veal flank steaks (about 3 flanks), or whole veal tenderloin

Preheat the oven to 375° F. Trim the meat of all visible fat and "silver skin."

Heat a seasoned sauté pan or a nonstick skillet and add one steak at a time. Sear for 2 minutes and turn. Each side should be well browned.

Repeat the process for each steak, letting the pan heat up before adding the meat.

Roast the flank steaks in a preheated 375° F oven for 5–6 minutes (10–12 minutes for a tenderloin roast). The centers should be pink.

Remove to a covered plate and let them rest for at least 5 minutes. Slice thinly against the grain.

SERVES 8

3 ounces per serving

	Fat (g)	Cholesterol (g)	Sodium (mg)	Calories
Total Recipe	34.4	837.6	2112	1056
Per Portion	4.3	104.7	264	132

Veal Flank with Rosemary and Garlic

This is a simple and flavorful way to prepare one of the lower-fat cuts of veal. The same method can be applied to other cuts or to beef or pork. Though veal is higher in cholesterol than other meats, it is lower in fat and calories. Although dried rosemary will do, try to use the fresh variety; it offers a great deal more aromatic flavor, which gives this recipe its zest.

3/4 **pound veal flank steak (1–2 steaks)**
2 **teaspoons minced fresh garlic**
4 **teaspoons fresh rosemary, chopped (or 4 teaspoons dried rosemary)**

Trim the meat of all visible fat and "silver skin." Dry the meat with a white paper towel and rub with the garlic.

Heat a large, heavy skillet over medium-high heat. When the pan is quite hot, sauté one steak at a time for 2–3 minutes on each side, creating a golden brown crust. Let the pan get hot before continuing to the second steak.

Remove the meat and lightly press half of the rosemary onto the top of the steaks. Next, broil the steaks for 3 minutes with the rosemary facing up. Turn them over and lightly press the remaining rosemary onto the meat. Broil for 3 more minutes. The centers should be pink.

Remove the meat to a platter and let it rest covered for at least 5 minutes before cutting. Slice the meat thinly at an angle against the grain.

SERVES 4
3 ounces per serving

	Fat (g)	Cholesterol (g)	Sodium (mg)	Calories
Total Recipe	17.2	418.8	1238	724
Per Portion	4.3	104.7	309	181

Coffee Milk Shake

This snack is for coffee ice cream lovers. It is nearly nonfat and extremely low in sodium. Try it as a snack or for a dessert drink.

1 cup Coffee Sauce (page 219)
1¹/₂ cups of ice
2 sprigs fresh mint, for garnish

Place the coffee sauce in the blender and add ice until it becomes smooth and frosty. Continue adding ice until it reaches desired consistency.

Serve with a sprig of fresh mint.

SERVES 2

	Fat (g)	Cholesterol (g)	Sodium (mg)	Calories
Total Recipe	2.2	0	28.2	61.2
Per Portion	1.1	0	14.1	30.6

Banana Coconut Freeze

This shake is very tropical and refreshing. When your overripe bananas accumulate, freeze them wrapped in plastic and save them for this recipe (or for baking). Try it with a teaspoon of wheat germ on top!

¹/₂ very ripe banana (frozen in plastic wrap without its skin)
¹/₂ cup nonfat plain yogurt
¹/₄ cup 2-percent or lowfat milk
1 teaspoon coconut extract
¹/₁₆ teaspoon freshly grated nutmeg (about 1 large pinch)

When the banana has partially defrosted, carefully slice it into ¹/₂-inch pieces. Blend the banana with the yogurt, milk, and coconut extract in a blender until smooth.

Top with the nutmeg and serve.

SERVES 2

	Fat (g)	Cholesterol (g)	Sodium (mg)	Calories
Total Recipe	14.8	0	89.8	247
Per Portion	7.4	0	44.9	123.5

— Fruit with Spiced Cream —

This cream is great with all kinds of fruit and can be used as a dessert dip or as a sauce. Or serve it whipped like a sweetened butter with Maple Breakfast Scones (page 100).

1/2 cup Thickest Yogurt (page 88)
2 teaspoons honey, or more to taste
1/16 teaspoon ground cardamom (about 1 large pinch)
1/16 teaspoon ground cinnamon (about 1 large pinch)
Fruit Salad (page 114)
1/4 cup sliced almonds

Stir the yogurt, honey, and spices together.

Roast the almonds on a baking sheet in a 350° F oven for 7–8 minutes, or until their aroma is released.

Serve the fruit salad and top each plate with a dollop of the yogurt mixture. Sprinkle with the almonds.

SERVES 4

	Fat (g)	Cholesterol (g)	Sodium (mg)	Calories
Total Recipe	33.2	0	620	976.8
Per Portion	8.3	0	155	244.2

— Spicy Peaches —

This nearly nonfat dessert is high in fiber yet very low in sodium and calories. It is also high in spice, creaminess, and the sweetness of fresh peaches. Use only very ripe, juicy, sweet peaches.

1 cup nonfat yogurt
1/4 teaspoon ground cinnamon
1 tablespoon chopped crystallized ginger
2 ripe peaches, sliced
1/2 teaspoon light brown sugar

Blend the yogurt, cinnamon, and ginger together.

In four attractive ramekins, layer 1/4 of the peaches and 1/4 of the yogurt, repeating the process until you are finished, ending up with the yogurt on top.

Sprinkle the top with brown sugar and refrigerate for at least one hour. The brown sugar will melt into the yogurt.

SERVES 4

	Fat (g)	Cholesterol (g)	Sodium (mg)	Calories
Total Recipe	.2	0	182.4	303.6
Per Portion	trace	0	45.6	75.9

Pears on a Raspberry Cloud

This dessert is very light in sugar for those who prefer a less sweet dessert. Though it lacks the sweetness, it offers subtle pear and raspberry flavors. It is low in calories and extremely low in fat and sodium. Serve it with a generous sprig of fresh mint.

> 2 cups water
> 1/4 cup sugar
> 2 cups Ariél brand dealcoholized premium white Zinfandel
>   wine
> 5 Bartlett pears, ripe and still firm
> 3 whole cloves
> 12 anise seeds, or 1 star anise, optional
> 1 1/2 teaspoons sugar
> 1 teaspoon raspberry flavor extract
> 12 raspberries, fresh or frozen without sugar and partially
>   thawed
> 2 tablespoons cold water
> 4 sprigs fresh mint for garnish

In a heavy, nonaluminum saucepan, heat the sugar and 1 cup of water over medium-high heat until the sugar melts. Add the remaining 1 cup of water, wine, cloves, and anise.

After washing the pears thoroughly, submerge them in the wine broth and bring them barely to a simmer. If they will not stay under the liquid, place a small lightweight plate on top to rest gently on the pears and hold them down. Reduce the heat to low.

Cook at low temperature for about 20 minutes or until an inserted sharp knife pulls out smoothly. Remove the pears from the broth and set aside or they will become too soft.

Chill the pears for at least 1 hour. Before serving, make the sauce by peeling and coring 1 pear. In a food processor fitted with a metal blade, blend the pear with the sugar, raspberry extract, raspberries, and cold water.

Carefully peel the remaining poached pears, preserving their shape. Halve and core them, and slice thinly.

Serve the pears well chilled. If more than a few minutes has passed since blending the sauce, process it again until slightly frothy. Place the pears on top of the sauce, which should rise up slightly to surround the pear like a cloud. Fresh mint is all you need.

SERVES 4

	Fat (g)	Cholesterol (g)	Sodium (mg)	Calories
Total Recipe	4	0	9.2	680
Per Portion	1	0	2.3	170

Tropical Fruits with Lime and Black Pepper

This refreshing and simple dessert is low in calories, while the sodium and fat contents are barely worth mentioning. Kiwi fruit and papaya are high in vitamin C.

1 ripe papaya
2 ripe kiwis
8 large red strawberries
juice of 2 limes
3/4 teaspoon cracked black pepper
4 lime wedges, optional

Peel, halve, and slice the papaya into four equal portions. Peel and slice the kiwi into 1/4-inch slices. After carefully washing the strawberries, cut them in half, leaving a portion of stem with each half.

Arrange the fruit on a decorative plate, lace with the cracked black pepper, and squeeze lime juice over all the fruit. You can also serve fresh lime with each portion.

SERVES 4

	Fat (g)	Cholesterol (g)	Sodium (mg)	Calories
Total Recipe	1.6	0	18.8	265.6
Per Portion	.4	0	4.7	66.4

Gingered Peaches

This is a luscious and intense dessert. Try to find white peaches, but yellow ones will do—the juicier, the better!

2 white (or yellow) peaches, ripe and juicy
4 slices angel food cake
2 tablespoons ginger preserves
1 1/2 tablespoons Ariél brand dealcoholized premium dry white wine
4 sprigs fresh mint for garnish

Mix the preserves with the wine until well blended.

Slice the peaches very thinly and fan them over the angel food cake.

Just before serving, carefully spoon the ginger sauce over the peaches, letting some of the sauce soak into the cake. Serve with fresh mint.

SERVES 4

	Fat (g)	Cholesterol (g)	Sodium (mg)	Calories
Total Recipe	.7	0	604	968
Per Portion	.17	0	151	242

Minted Honeydew with "Champagne"

This dessert is elegant, refreshing, and full of surprising flavors. The touch of champagne really makes a difference in taste and in appeal. Always use fresh mint.

4 cups honeydew melon balls
1/2 cup fresh blueberries
4 tablespoons mint, sliced finely
6 ounces Ariél brand dealcoholized premium brut
     "champagne"

Use your most decorative bowls. Arrange the melon balls and sprinkle with the berries and then the mint.

You can add the champagne at the table if you wish. It will bubble up around the fruit.

SERVES 4

	Fat (g)	Cholesterol (g)	Sodium (mg)	Calories
Total Recipe	.8	0	80.4	420
Per Portion	.2	0	20.1	105

– Grapes with "Sour Cream" – and Brown Sugar

This is a revision of a classic dessert, this time with much less fat and fewer calories. You can't predict the flavors until you try it; it's sweet and rich and refreshing.

1/4 **cup nondairy sour cream**
3/4 **cup nonfat plain yogurt**
1/2 **cup seedless red grapes, chilled**
1/2 **cup seedless green grapes, chilled**
4 **teaspoons light brown sugar**

In a small bowl, blend the sour cream and yogurt until creamy.

Fold the grapes and sour cream together and spoon into four dessert dishes. Refrigerate until serving.

Just before serving, sprinkle the brown sugar evenly over each of the bowls.

SERVES 4

	Fat (g)	Cholesterol (g)	Sodium (mg)	Calories
Total Recipe	12	0	156	377.6
Per Portion	3	0	39	94.4

Crisped Blueberries with "Sour Cream"

This dessert can be made with very thinly sliced apples and pears or with bananas. It is lower in fat, sodium, and calories than most fruit crisps and is high in fiber. The crisp is sweet and fruity, while the "sour cream" topping adds a tart richness.

vegetable oil spray
1 pint fresh blueberries
1 cup quick-cooking rolled oats
1 teaspoon vanilla extract
1/4 cup loosely packed light brown sugar
1 tablespoon unsalted margarine
1 egg white, beaten
1/4 teaspoon ground cinnamon
4 teaspoons Thickest Yogurt (page 88)
4 fresh mint sprigs for garnish

Use a nonstick baking dish or spray a baking dish with vegetable oil spray before putting the blueberries in.

Heat a small saucepan over medium heat and melt the sugar, spices, vanilla, and margarine. Add the oats to this mixture and stir. Use a spatula to remove all of the sugar sauce from the pan in the next step.

Spread the crisp mixture over the fruit and bake in a 350° F oven for 15–20 minutes on a top shelf of the oven. The fruit should be cooked and soft but still intact and the oats lightly browned.

Stir the yogurt until smooth and light and drop a spoonful on the warm crisp before serving. Serve with fresh mint.

SERVES 4

	Fat (g)	Cholesterol (g)	Sodium (mg)	Calories
Total Recipe	10	0	199.2	581.2
Per Portion	2.5	0	49.8	145.3

Strawberry Trifle

This version of trifle is sweet and satisfying with strawberries. Trifle is usually rich with fatty creams, but this one avoids the fat altogether. It is sweet, so a little goes a long way.

**1¹/2 cups strawberries, fresh or frozen without sugar and
  partially thawed**
2 tablespoons sugar, or to taste
**2 tablespoons Ariél brand dealcoholized premium dry white
  wine**
3 tablespoons fresh lemon or lime juice

1 cup Thickest Yogurt (page 88)
**4 tablespoons Ariél brand dealcoholized premium dry white
  wine**
4 tablespoons all-fruit strawberry preserves
2 teaspoons strawberry or raspberry flavor extract
3/4 of a 9-inch angel food cake, 8 slices
1 pint fresh sweet strawberries

In a food processor fitted with a metal blade, purée the first group of ingredients: berries, sugar, wine, and lemon or lime juice. Set the sauce aside.

In a small bowl, mix the yogurt, wine, preserves, and berry extract until smooth.

Slice the cake thinly. In a decorative bowl, layer 1/3 of the cake and top with 1/2 of the strawberry sauce. Continue layering until finished. Spread the yogurt cream on top.

Refrigerate for at least one hour. Decorate the top and/or sides generously with the fresh berries.

SERVES 8

	Fat (g)	Cholesterol (g)	Sodium (mg)	Calories
Total Recipe	3.1	0	1403	931
Per Portion	.4	0	175.4	241.4

Raspberry Turnovers

The flaky filo dough punches all the right buttons for pastry lovers. Serve it with Mango Sauce (page 218).

1 tablespoon unsalted margarine
1/2 cup Thickest Yogurt (page 88)
2 tablespoons raspberry preserves (fruit-only type)
2 sheets filo dough
1 pint sweet raspberries

Melt the margarine in a small pan and set aside. In a small bowl, blend the yogurt and the preserves. If the raspberries are tart, add a little sugar to the yogurt mixture.

Defrost the filo dough as prescribed on the box and remove two sheets. Lay them out and cut in half.

Carefully brush a small amount of melted margarine onto 2 of the halves and place the other two halves on top.

With kitchen scissors, cut the 2 double sheets in half once again, creating 4 double sheets.

Place 1/4 of the raspberries just below and to the left of center of each piece and top with the raspberry and yogurt mixture.

Carefully fold the lower right corner over the raspberries, making a triangle. Fold this triangle up and continue folding to the right to make a triangular "football." Or, place the raspberries and sauce in the center of the sheet and simply wrap the dough around it, crimping it in at the center, like a piece of candy.

Lightly brush the exposed top of the turnover with the remaining melted margarine.

Preheat the oven to 375° F and bake for about 8 minutes or until golden.

SERVES 4

	Fat (g)	Cholesterol (g)	Sodium (mg)	Calories
Total Recipe	8	0	160	408
Per Portion	2	0	40	102

Apple Crisp

This dish can be served as a dessert as is or with frozen nonfat yogurt or for a breakfast side dish with yogurt or a little cold, low-fat milk poured over it.

vegetable oil spray
6 Granny Smith apples, peeled and chopped
1¹/₂ teaspoons ground cinnamon
2 tablespoons lemon juice
2 teaspoons sugar
¹/₂ cup quick-cooking oats
¹/₄ cup toasted wheat germ
2 tablespoons packed brown sugar
¹/₄ cup orange or apple juice

Spray a large, heavy skillet with vegetable spray. Heat over medium-high heat and when a few drops of water sizzle, add the apples and reduce the heat to medium.

Cook the apples, stirring occasionally. After about 10 minutes add ¹/₂ teaspoon cinnamon; after 25 minutes add the lemon juice and sugar. Remove the apples from the heat when they are soft, but not mushy.

Preheat the oven to 350° F. In a small bowl, mix the oats, wheat germ, 1 teaspoon cinnamon, and brown sugar.

Put the cooked apples in a baking dish or in 6 ramekins. Top with the crumb mixture and drizzle the juice over top.

Bake at 350° F for about 25 minutes.

SERVES 6

	Fat (g)	Cholesterol (g)	Sodium (mg)	Calories
Total Recipe	10.2	0	17.4	953.4
Per Portion	1.7	0	2.9	158.9

— Mocha Almond Pudding —

This is a rich-tasting dessert and has all the allure of more fatty desserts, such as mocha flavoring, cake, and nuts. I like the free-form appearance that invites tasting with large spoons. If you like a more formal presentation, use a small springform tart pan or a crystal bowl. The recipe calls for champagne biscuits, which are the crisp Italian version of ladyfingers. They can be found in gourmet markets if your supermarket doesn't carry imported items. Or they can be created by simply letting ladyfingers dry out. This recipe can easily be doubled or tripled.

1 cup nonfat vanilla yogurt
3/4 cup freshly brewed decaffeinated coffee
3 teaspoons instant decaffeinated coffee or espresso
1 tablespoon sugar
2 teaspoons chocolate flavor extract
5 champagne biscuits or dry ladyfingers
2 tablespoons sliced almonds
1 tablespoon bittersweet chocolate shavings

The night before, thicken the yogurt as in Thickest Yogurt (page 88). Prepare the almonds by roasting them on a baking sheet in a 350° F oven for 7–8 minutes, or until their aroma is released. Keep a close watch so they don't burn.

When the yogurt is ready, brew the coffee on the strong side and stir in the instant coffee and sugar. Let the mixture cool until it is room temperature and stir in the chocolate extract.

Dip three biscuits or dry ladyfingers in the coffee mixture just long enough to soak them so that they absorb the coffee mixture but don't drip; they should remain intact. Place them in the center of a decorative plate.

Spread half of the thickened yogurt carefully on the biscuits. Soak two more biscuits as above and place them in the center of the first three, like a pyramid.

Top with the remaining yogurt. Sprinkle the chocolate shavings on the top. Press the almonds into the pudding around the top edge; taking a few at a time, lightly insert them and let go so they stick out.

This pudding is delicious alone or served with Coffee Sauce (page 219).

SERVES 4

	Fat (g)	Cholesterol (g)	Sodium (mg)	Calories
Total Recipe	35.7	5	260.25	1048.5
Per Portion	8.9	1.3	65.1	262.1

- Lemon Strawberry Pudding -

This pudding tastes as rich as it is low in fat and calories. It is fairly low in sodium and very low in cholesterol. The strawberries provide a good source of vitamin C. Champagne biscuits are the Italian version of ladyfingers and are crisp; they can be found in gourmet markets if your supermarket doesn't carry imported items. Or they can be created simply by letting ladyfingers dry out.

1 cup nonfat lemon yogurt
1 cup fresh strawberries (the ripest ones you have)
1 tablespoon sugar, or to taste
3 champagne biscuits, or dry ladyfingers
1 recipe Strawberry Sauce (page 218)

The night before, thicken the yogurt as in Thickest Yogurt (page 88).
Slice the strawberries, sprinkle them with the sugar, and toss gently.
Layer the biscuits or ladyfingers in a small decorative bowl and spoon a few spoonfuls of the sauce over them. Cover with the berries.
Spread the thick lemon yogurt over the berries and refrigerate until chilled.
Top with Strawberry Sauce and garnish with fresh mint.
SERVES 2

	Fat (g)	Cholesterol (g)	Sodium (mg)	Calories
Total Recipe	2.4	47.2	190.2	582
Per Portion	1.2	23.6	95.1	291

Vanilla Almond Pudding

This is very creamy, for those who like whipped cream toppings on cake. For a dessert this rich-tasting, it is low in fat and calories, and fairly low in sodium. It has no cholesterol. Serve the pudding with Blueberry Sauce (page 217).

4 cups nonfat vanilla yogurt
4 slices angel food cake, about 1/2-inch thick
1 teaspoon almond extract
1/2 cup sliced almonds, roasted

Overnight, thicken the vanilla yogurt as in Thickest Yogurt (page 88).

When the yogurt is ready, cover the bottom of a 6-inch crock or small baking dish with slices of angel food cake.

Roughly chop the roasted almonds, either by hand or in the food processor. Don't let them pulverize completely.

Mix the thickened yogurt with the almond extract and spread over the cake. Top with the almonds.

Serve the pudding alone, or with Blueberry Sauce (page 217).

SERVES 4

	Fat (g)	Cholesterol (g)	Sodium (mg)	Calories
Total Recipe	29.2	0	760	1256
Per Portion	7.3	0	190	314

—— Baked Spiced Bananas ——

These bananas are great for breakfast with milk poured over them or as a side dish with black beans. Try serving them with Curried Black Beans (page 109) or Black Beans with Orange and Jalapeño (page 108). Since the pan drippings resemble melted butter, they can be spooned over nonfat vanilla frozen yogurt and topped with just a pinch of coconut for a seemingly sinful dessert. (One half teaspoon of shredded coconut has only .6 milligrams of fat.)

4 bananas, ripe and firm
1/4 cup light brown sugar
1 teaspoon ground cinnamon
1/4 teaspoon ground cardamom
2 tablespoons fresh lemon juice

Preheat the oven to 375° F. In a small bowl, combine the brown sugar and spices. Using a nonstick baking sheet or a medium baking pan sprayed with vegetable oil spray, place the bananas close together on the pan.

Slice the bananas lengthwise and gently press the brown sugar mixture onto the top of each. Drizzle the lemon juice over each mound of sugar.

Bake at 375° F until the sugar starts to bubble.

Pour the pan drippings over the bananas before serving.

SERVES 4

	Fat (g)	Cholesterol (g)	Sodium (mg)	Calories
Total Recipe	2.52	0	20.96	640
Per Portion	.63	0	5.24	160

Spiced Pears with Almond Chips

This pear dessert is low in calories and fat. It is especially enjoyable around the winter holiday because it fills the house with beautiful spicy smells. It also makes a great snack with nonfat yogurt, or even nonfat frozen yogurt.

juice and grated rind of 1 orange, no white pulp
1 lemon, sliced
2 inches fresh ginger root, peeled and sliced
6 firm pears
12 whole cloves
3 cinnamon sticks
2 tablespoons curry powder
1 cup sugar
8 cups water, or to cover
2 star anise
1/2 cup sliced almonds
2 tablespoons cornstarch
2 tablespoons cold water

In a nonaluminum pan, combine all the ingredients except the almonds, cornstarch, and cold water. Heat to a low simmer. Cook for 1 hour or until the pears are tender but still firm.

Meanwhile, roast the almonds on a nonstick baking sheet at 350° F for 5–7 minutes, or until their aroma is released and they just begin to turn golden.

When the pears are tender yet firm, remove them from the pan and let them cool slightly.

Meanwhile, continue cooking the poaching liquid until reduced to approximately 2 1/2 cups.

In a small bowl or glass, combine the cold water and corn starch and slowly stir into the hot syrup. Cook 5 minutes longer.

To prepare for serving, halve, core, and slice the pears. Arrange in baking dish, cover with syrup and set aside until ready to reheat.

Heat in 350° F preheated oven for approximately 1 hour, or until hot and tender.

Serve with the reduced sauce, and dust with roasted slivered almonds.

SERVES 12
1/2 pear per serving

	Fat (g)	Cholesterol (g)	Sodium (mg)	Calories
Total Recipe	63.6	0	885.6	2112
Per Portion	5.3	0	73.8	176

Blueberry Sauce

This is a cool and refreshing dessert sauce that is nonfat. It's also very low in sodium and calories; it also happens to be high in fiber. Serve it with Vanilla Almond Pudding (page 214), or over frozen yogurt or fresh fruit.

1 cup fresh blueberries
1 cup chopped honeydew melon
1/8 teaspoon ground cardamom (about 2 pinches)
1/8 teaspoon ground nutmeg (about 2 pinches)
2 teaspoons sugar, or to taste

Blend all the ingredients in a blender or food processor. If it is too thick for your liking, add a little water.

If you refrigerate it before serving, you may find that it solidifies. If so, reblend it right before serving.

Garnish with fresh mint sprigs.

SERVES 6
1/3 cup per serving

	Fat (g)	Cholesterol (g)	Sodium (mg)	Calories
Total Recipe	1.2	0	25.2	114.4
Per Portion	.2	0	4.2	28.6

Strawberry Sauce

This sauce is a good source of vitamin C, with almost no fat and sodium. It is extremely versatile; serve it with Lemon Strawberry Pudding (page 213) or with any display of fresh exotic fruits.

> 1 cup fresh, or frozen defrosted, strawberries (no sugar added)
> 1/4 cup Ariél brand dealcoholized premium dry white wine
> 1 tablespoon sugar or to taste

B lend the ingredients in a blender and serve cold. Add sugar to taste if necessary, depending on the ripeness of the berries.

Serve well chilled.

SERVES 2

	Fat (g)	Cholesterol (g)	Sodium (mg)	Calories
Total Recipe	.8	0	6.2	252
Per Portion	.2	0	3.1	126

Mango Sauce

Find a fully ripe mango and you will have a naturally sweet, low-fat, low-sodium, and very rich dessert sauce. Try it with fruits or frozen yogurt to create a soothing, tropical effect. Adjust the ingredients depending upon the sweetness of the fruit. Try it with a pinch of ground cinnamon.

> 1 ripe mango
> 2 teaspoons sugar
> 1 teaspoon Ariél brand dealcoholized premium dry white wine
> 2 teaspoons water

W ith a paring knife, cut the mango away from its large center core by cutting from top to bottom in several sections. Remove the skin from these sections and trim any remaining fruit from the core, catching the juices as you go.

In a food processor fitted with a metal blade, purée the fruit until smooth.

Add the remaining ingredients and blend until pourable. Add additional water or wine if you need to thin the sauce. If the fruit lacks sweetness, add sugar to taste.

SERVES 8

	Fat (g)	Cholesterol (g)	Sodium (mg)	Calories
Total Recipe	.6	0	4.8	160
Per Portion	trace	0	.6	20

Coffee Sauce

This dessert sauce is very intense in flavor, yet very low in fat! It can accompany any pudding, frozen yogurt, or fresh fruit. Or, save the leftovers for a Coffee Milk Shake (page 201).

¹/₂ cup water
2 tablespoons instant decaffeinated coffee or espresso
4 tablespoons sugar
2 teaspoons chocolate flavor extract
1 cup nonfat plain yogurt

Boil the water. Remove from the heat and stir in the instant coffee, sugar, and chocolate extract.

Let the mixture cool and stir in the yogurt until smooth.

Refrigerate the sauce until very cold.

SERVES 8

	Fat (g)	Cholesterol (g)	Sodium (mg)	Calories
Total Recipe	8	0	197.6	428
Per Portion	1	0	24.7	53.5

Spiced Fruit Sauce

This can be served as a sauce under a display of fresh fruit, as a fruit dip, or with scones instead of butter or cream. It is low in sodium and fat, but high in flavor. Its thick and creamy texture tastes as rich as a sour cream sauce.

1/2 cup Thickest Yogurt (page 88)
2 dates, minced
1 teaspoon rum flavor extract
1 tablespoon fig preserves (or orange marmalade)
1/16 teaspoon freshly ground nutmeg (about 1 large pinch)

Stir the ingredients together until smooth. Let the sauce rest in the refrigerator for 1 hour and adjust the flavorings to suit your taste. If necessary, add a little water to thin the sauce, depending upon your use.

Whip with a spoon before serving.

SERVES 4

	Fat (g)	Cholesterol (g)	Sodium (mg)	Calories
Total Recipe	.3	0	3.6	216
Per Portion	trace	0	.9	54

— Currant and Yam Scones —

These scones are lower in sodium than many scones, since they use baking powder instead of soda and offer the beta-carotene of yams. While scones can be enjoyed for breakfast or for tea, this recipe makes an interesting sandwich, since it is only slightly sweet.

1 tablespoon water
1 teaspoon rum flavor extract
2 tablespoons currants (or raisins)
2 teaspoons baking powder
1 teaspoon ground ginger
1/2 teaspoon ground nutmeg
1 cup well cooked yam (about 1 medium yam, peeled and
   mashed)
1 tablespoon unsalted margarine, melted
1 tablespoon sugar
2 tablespoons water
1 cup unbleached all-purpose flour
1 egg white, beaten with 1 teaspoon water

Preheat the oven to 375° F. In a small bowl, soak the currants in the water and rum flavor while you work. Sift the flour, baking powder, ginger, and nutmeg together into a large bowl.

In a food processor fitted with a metal blade, purée the potatoes while warm or at room temperature, whichever is more convenient. Add the melted shortening and sugar and blend.

Blend the water into the yam mixture and stir in the flour in three installments. If using the food processor, pulse the blade rather than letting it run. Over-handling will produce a tough dough.

When the dough pulls away from the sides of the bowl or food processor, remove it to a lightly floured surface. Give the dough a few gentle kneads to bring it together.

Form the dough into a round about 1/2-inch thick. A large scone is handy for sandwich wedges or for splitting and toasting. You can also create individual scones of any size for serving with tea. The surface of the dough should be relatively smooth. Place the scone on a nonstick baking sheet or one sprayed with vegetable oil spray.

Remove the currants from the rum flavor and gently press them into the top of the scone. Brush the top and sides lightly with the egg white wash.

Bake at 375° F for 20–25 minutes. The crust should just begin to brown.

SERVES 6

1 wedge or 2 small scones per serving

	Fat (g)	Cholesterol (g)	Sodium (mg)	Calories
Total Recipe	9.6	0	957.6	677.4
Per Portion	1.6	0	159.6	112.9

— Southwestern Corn Bread —

This corn bread is lower in fat and sodium than many corn breads, but the addition of cilantro and corn kernels makes it unique.

1¹/2 cups yellow cornmeal
1/2 cup unbleached all-purpose flour
3 teaspoons baking powder
1 egg, beaten
1 cup skim milk
1 tablespoon packed light brown sugar
1 teaspoon Cilantro Pesto (page 94)
1 cup cooked corn kernels; frozen, defrosted corn; or
    kernels from 1 ear of freshly cooked corn
vegetable oil spray

In a large bowl combine the dry ingredients. Preheat the oven to 425° F.

Strain the corn from any liquid it might be in.

In a small bowl combine the egg, milk, brown sugar, and Cilantro Pesto. With a large spatula or spoon, add this mixture and the corn to the dry ingredients. Blend in a few strokes.

Spray a 9-by-9-inch baking pan with vegetable oil spray. Fill with the batter and bake for about 20 minutes, or until golden on top.

SERVES 9

	Fat (g)	Cholesterol (g)	Sodium (mg)	Calories
Total Recipe	11.7	278.1	1509.3	783
Per Portion	1.3	30.9	167.7	87

Crusty Italian Bread

Almost nonexistent fat and sodium and no cholesterol make this bread a low-calorie splurge. Save leftover bread, let it dry out, and make your own low-sodium bread crumbs. If you choose to add the salt, just add 125 milligrams of sodium to each serving.

1 package active dry yeast (1 tablespoon)
1½ cups warm water (110° F–115° F)
1 teaspoon sugar
½ teaspoon salt (optional)
1 tablespoon olive oil
3¾ cups unbleached all-purpose flour
4 tablespoons wheat germ
½ teaspoon dried thyme leaves
¼ teaspoon dried oregano leaves

In a large bowl, dissolve the yeast and sugar thoroughly with ½ cup of the water and let rest until small bubbles appear, about 10 minutes. If using a mixer with paddle and dough hook, this can be mixed in the mixer bowl.

In another bowl, combine the flour with the wheat germ and salt, if salt is desired.

Add the remaining water to the yeast mixture and begin to stir in the flour mixture with a wooden spoon. If using a mixer, use the paddle. Add the flour one cup at a time and stop adding flour when the mixture pulls away from the sides of the bowl and is a workable mass.

Empty onto a lightly floured surface and knead for approximately 8–10 minutes, dusting with the flour if the mass becomes sticky. If using a mixer, replace the paddle with the dough hook and knead for 3–5 minutes.

Stop kneading when the dough is soft and elastic, like the consistency of an ear lobe.

Form a smooth ball with the dough and place in a slightly oiled bowl and turn to coat all sides. Cover with a towel and let rise in a warm place for approximately 1 hour, or until doubled in size.

Punch the dough down, empty it onto a lightly floured surface and knead by hand a few times. Reform the dough into a ball and return it to the bowl. Turn the dough to coat with oil. Let it rise once more, about 1 hour, or until doubled in size.

Preheat the oven to 425° F. Turn the dough onto a lightly floured surface, knead it a few times, and shape into two smooth oblong loaves or one larger loaf. Sprinkle them with the herbs.

Bake the bread on a nonstick baking sheet. After placing it in a hot oven, cook for five minutes and reduce the oven to 375° F. Cook for 30–35 minutes, or until golden brown. The bread is cooked thoroughly when thumping the bottom of the loaf produces a hollow sound.

SERVES 10
1 slice per serving

	Fat (g)	Cholesterol (g)	Sodium (mg)	Calories
Total Recipe	25	0	14	1910
Per Portion	2.5	0	1.4	191

— Focaccia with Fresh Sage —

Focaccia is an Italian flatbread that is baked with olive oil, herbs, and salt. It can satisfy a pizza craving, hold an overstuffed sandwich, or accompany dinner. This version is low in sodium and lower in fat than traditional focaccia. The olive oil leaves little need for butter.

1 package active dry yeast (1 tablespoon)
1 1/2 cups warm water (110° F–115° F)
1 teaspoon sugar
3 cups unbleached, all-purpose flour
3/4 cup rye or whole wheat flour
4 tablespoons wheat germ
6 sage leaves, sliced thinly
1 tablespoon extra virgin olive oil

In a large bowl dissolve the yeast and sugar thoroughly with 1/2 cup of the water and let rest until small bubbles appear, about 10 minutes.

In another bowl, combine the all-purpose and rye or whole wheat flours with the wheat germ. Mix well.

Add the remaining water to the yeast mixture and stir. Add 1 cup of the flour mixture and stir well, using the paddle of a mixer, or a wooden spoon. Stir in one more cup of the flour mixture. Stir in the remaining flour mixture 1/2 cup at a time; stop adding flour when the mixture pulls away from the sides of the bowl and is a workable mass. If there is extra flour, reserve it.

Empty the dough onto a lightly floured surface if kneading by hand, or put the dough hook on the mixer. Knead for approximately 8–10 minutes by hand or for 3–5 minutes using the mixer, dusting with flour if the mass becomes sticky.

Stop kneading when the dough is soft and elastic, like the consistency of an ear lobe.

Form a smooth ball with the dough, place in a slightly oiled bowl and turn to coat all sides. Cover with a towel and let rise in a warm place for approximately 1 hour or until doubled in size.

Punch the dough down, knead it a few times, and roll it out into a 1/2-inch disk. Press your fingers down into the dough, making indentations.

Drizzle the olive oil over the top evenly and cover with the sage. Preheat the oven to 400° F.

Let the dough rest for about 20 minutes and bake at 400° F for 20–25 minutes or until golden brown. The bread is cooked thoroughly when thumping the bottom of the loaf produces a hollow sound.

SERVES 8

1 wedge per serving

	Fat (g)	Cholesterol (g)	Sodium (mg)	Calories
Total Recipe	21.6	0	11.2	1712
Per Portion	2.7	0	1.4	214

Gingered Rolls

Because they have just a hint of sweetness, these rolls can be served at breakfast, with tea, or with dinner. If you can't find ginger preserves, you might try making orange rolls with orange marmalade instead. Also, if you have a surplus of rolls, you might use them for Pineapple and Ham Ginger Biscuits (page 234).

1 package active dry yeast (1 tablespoon)
1¼ cups warm water (110° F–115° F)
¼ teaspoon sugar
2 tablespoons ginger preserves or orange marmalade
4 cups unbleached, all-purpose flour
1½ teaspoons fennel seed
2 teaspoons cinnamon
1 egg white, beaten with 1 teaspoon water

In a large bowl or the bowl of a food processor fitted with a kneading blade, thoroughly dissolve the yeast and sugar in 1/2 cup of warm water and let rest until small bubbles appear, about 10 minutes.

If the ginger pieces are large chop them up. Add the remaining 3/4 cup of water and the ginger preserves to the yeast mixture and stir to blend.

In another large bowl, stir together the flour, fennel seed, and cinnamon. Slowly stir the flour mixture into the yeast mixture with a wooden spoon, 1/2 cup at a time, until the dough starts to pull away from the bowl. If using the food processor, pulse the kneading blade to slowly add the flour.

In the food processor, knead the dough for 20–25 long pulses. (If using the food processor, knead the dough by hand for about a minute at the end.) Or turn the dough onto a lightly floured surface and knead it by hand for 10–15 minutes. If the dough sticks to your fingers, dust it with a little flour. Too much flour will make the dough hard to manage and tough to eat. The dough should be smooth, elastic, and supple, about the consistency of your ear lobe.

Form the dough into a smooth ball, place it in a large oiled bowl, and turn to coat all sides. Cover the dough and let it rise in a warm place for about an hour, or until it has doubled in volume.

Punch the dough down, turn it out onto a lightly floured surface, and knead it for 2–3 minutes further.

Spray two cake pans or one baking sheet with vegetable oil spray or use nonstick pans. Shape the dough into 12 small balls and place them on the pan, smooth side up. Let them rise for about 45 minutes.

Brush them with the egg white wash and bake at 375° F for about 30 minutes. The rolls should be golden brown and hollow sounding when thumped at their center underside.

SERVES 12
1 roll per serving

	Fat (g)	Cholesterol (g)	Sodium (mg)	Calories
Total Recipe	19.2	0	66	1884
Per Portion	1.6	0	5.5	157

Vegetarian Pizza

Try this as a snack or for a main course. It is very flavorful and rich in vitamin C. The vegetables, fresh rosemary, and Parmesan cheese give it aromatic power. Use the best quality imported Parmesan cheese you can find; it will make a difference.

½ recipe Pizza Dough (page 93)
½ small red pepper
½ small yellow pepper
3 green onions, dark green portion removed
1–2 cloves of elephant garlic
1 tablespoon fresh rosemary, chopped (or 2 teaspoons dried rosemary)
1 teaspoon extra virgin olive oil
2 tablespoons fresh grated Parmesan cheese

Roast the peppers under the broiler skin side up until the skin is dark and blistered. If you aren't a real garlic lover, roast the whole garlic clove with the peppers before the next step; pre-roasting it will reduce its pungency. The roasted garlic should not turn brown. Remove the peppers to a plastic bag and let them cool. When they cool peel the skin off, remove the seeds, and slice very thinly.

Quarter the green onions lengthwise, cut off the stem, and cut into 1-inch pieces. With a very sharp knife cut the garlic in half, turn the flat side down, and slice paper thin. Preheat the oven to 425° F.

On a lightly floured surface, roll the pizza dough out to about ¼-inch. Place it on a nonstick baking sheet. Spread the peppers over the dough first, then the garlic slices, onion, and rosemary. Drizzle with the olive oil.

Bake in a 425° F oven on the top shelf for 10 minutes. Transfer the pizza to the bottom shelf for 10 more minutes. In the last 2–3 minutes sprinkle the Parmesan cheese over the pizza.

SERVES 4
4 large pieces per serving

	Fat (g)	Cholesterol (g)	Sodium (mg)	Calories
Total Recipe	21.6	11.2	274.4	1102
Per Portion	5.4	2.8	68.6	275.5

– White Pizza with Rosemary –

There is no need to deprive yourself of pizza. This white pizza is both cheesy and robust, while low in fat, calories, and sodium. The portions below are for a snack or appetizer. You can't go wrong even if you decide to double up. If you want to use salt in the cheese recipe, just add 64 milligrams of sodium per serving.

1/2 **package dry yeast (1¹/2 teaspoons)**
3/4 **cups warm water**
1/2 **teaspoon sugar**
1/4 **teaspoon salt (optional)**
1 **tablespoon olive oil**
1 3/4 **cups flour**
2 **tablespoons wheat germ**
1/2 **recipe Herbed Ricotta Cheese (page 233)**

In a large bowl, dissolve the yeast and sugar thoroughly with 1/2 cup of the water and let rest until small bubbles appear, about 10 minutes. If using a mixer with paddle and dough hook, this can be mixed in the mixer bowl.

In another bowl, combine the flour with the wheat germ and salt, if salt is desired.

Add the remaining water and olive oil to the yeast mixture and begin to stir in the flour mixture with a wooden spoon. If using a mixer, use the paddle. Add the flour one cup at a time and stop adding flour when the mixture pulls away from the sides of the bowl and is a workable mass.

Empty onto a lightly floured surface and knead for approximately 8–10 minutes, dusting with the flour if the mass becomes sticky. If using a mixer, replace the paddle with the dough hook and knead for 3–5 minutes.

Stop kneading when the dough is soft and elastic, like the consistency of an ear lobe.

Form a smooth ball with the dough, place it in a slightly oiled bowl, and turn to coat all sides. Cover with a towel and let rise in a warm place for approximately 1 hour, or until doubled in size.

Working on a lightly floured surface, form the dough into 12 balls and roll into 12 4-inch circles.

Cover each with one tablespoon of the Herbed Ricotta Cheese mixture.

Place six pizzas each on 2 baking sheets sprayed with vegetable oil spray.

Bake in a 425° F preheated oven, placing one pan on the center rack and the other pan on a rack below center of the oven. After 8 minutes reverse the pans and cook for 8 more minutes.

SERVES 6
2 miniature pizzas per serving

	Fat (g)	Cholesterol (g)	Sodium (mg)	Calories
Total Recipe	32.4	75.6	228.6	1663.6
Per Portion	5.4	12.6	38.1	218

Garlic Bread with Tomatoes and Herbs

This garlic bread is low in sodium and calories, especially if you use Crusty Italian Bread (page 223). The fat that it does provide is from olive oil, high in monounsaturates. If you would like to lower the fat content of this dish, simply reduce the amount of olive oil used to flavor the toast. Serve this as an appetizer or as a light lunch with a vegetable salad. With the sweetness of the tomato and the aromatics of the oregano, salt is unnecessary.

> 1 **medium vine-ripened tomato or 1 cup ripe plum tomatoes, chopped**
> 2 **teaspoons fresh garlic, minced**
> 2 **tablespoons extra virgin olive oil**
> 1 **teaspoon chopped fresh oregano or scant ¼ teaspoon dried oregano**
> 1 **tablespoon balsamic vinegar**
> 1 **teaspoon extra virgin olive oil**
> ½ **teaspoon coarse black pepper**
> 4 **thick slices of Italian bread, cut ¾ inch thick**

Dice the tomato in uniform ¼-inch cubes and let them rest in a sieve for about 15 minutes, allowing the water to drain off.

Warm two teaspoons of minced garlic and 2 tablespoons olive oil in a small pan. *Do not* brown the garlic, but allow it to cook slowly for 2–3 minutes. Remove from the heat.

In a bowl, combine the tomato, oregano, 1 teaspoon olive oil, vinegar, and black pepper. Set aside at room temperature.

Toast the Italian bread on both sides and brush with the garlic and olive oil mixture.

When ready to serve, put the toast under the broiler or toaster oven for about 2 minutes to reheat; spoon the tomato mixture over the top.

SERVES 4

	Fat (g)	Cholesterol (g)	Sodium (mg)	Calories
Total Recipe	41.2	0	18	1075.2
Per Portion	10.3	0	4.5	268.8

Garlic Toast with White Beans

This treat can serve as an appetizer before a light meal or for lunch with a vegetable salad. It is low in fat and sodium, yet satisfying and flavorful.

1 teaspoon extra virgin olive oil
2 teaspoons fresh garlic, minced
1/2 cup dry white beans
1/4 teaspoon red pepper flakes
2 teaspoons dried rosemary
1/4 bay leaf
3 1/2 cups Low-Sodium Chicken Stock (page 88)
2 teaspoons extra virgin olive oil
1 teaspoon fresh garlic, minced
4 slices Crusty Italian Bread (page 223) or other Italian
  bread, cut into 3/4-inch slices

In a medium, heavy saucepan, heat the olive oil over medium heat. Add the garlic and sauté for about 5 minutes until soft; do not brown.

Stir in the beans and coat them with the oil. Add the pepper, rosemary, bay leaf, and chicken stock and bring to a low simmer.

Cook uncovered about 1 1/4 hours until the beans are tender but not mushy. If too much liquid evaporates and the beans begin to rise above the stock, add a little water. When done, cover them and let rest about 30 minutes.

Meanwhile, heat 2 teaspoons of olive oil in a small pan over medium heat and cook the garlic slowly; do not brown.

Toast the Italian bread and brush with the garlic and olive oil.

Remove and discard the bay leaf and spoon the hot beans over the toast just before serving.

SERVES 4

	Fat (g)	Cholesterol (g)	Sodium (mg)	Calories
Total Recipe	30.8	0	297.6	1451.6
Per Portion	7.7	0	74.4	362.9

Apricots with Goat Cheese and Sage

These apricots make a great appetizer or an accompaniment to a salad for lunch. Ask your local gourmet market if they carry a low-fat variety of goat cheese; otherwise, use regular goat cheese. This will add 2 grams of fat per serving.

> **4 fresh ripe apricots, split**
> **1/2 piece of imported, extra lean ham, rinsed with cold water and cut into 1-by-1/16-inch pieces**
> **6 fresh sage leaves, cut 1/16-inch thin**
> **1 ounce low-fat goat cheese**
> **2 tablespoons Thickest Yogurt (page 88)**

In a small bowl, blend the yogurt and goat cheese until very creamy.

Spread the cheese mixture on each of the apricot halves, leaving a border of apricot exposed.

Place a small amount of ham matchsticks randomly on each piece of fruit.

Broil the halves for about 2 minutes, 2 inches from the element, just before serving. The cheese will warm and the ham will start to brown. Top with the sage and continue broiling for a moment to release its aroma.

SERVES 4
2 pieces per serving

	Fat (g)	Cholesterol (g)	Sodium (mg)	Calories
Total Recipe	3.6	8	282.8	157.2
Per Portion	.9	2	70.7	39.3

Sesame Dip

This dip is very low in sodium and fat and has all the flavor you might want for cold vegetables or toasted pita bread. It also makes a great spread or dressing for sandwiches. This freezes well; defrost overnight in the refrigerator and blend well before serving.

4 ounces soft tofu
1¹/₂ teaspoons minced garlic
1¹/₂ teaspoons grated ginger root
¹/₈ teaspoon ground white pepper (about 2 pinches)
¹/₁₆ teaspoon cayenne pepper (about 1 pinch)
¹/₄ cup nonfat plain yogurt
1 tablespoon plus 1 teaspoon tahini (sesame paste)
¹/₄ teaspoon sesame oil, or to taste
1 tablespoon freshly squeezed lime or lemon juice
1 teaspoon chopped fresh cilantro, or 1 tablespoon chopped
 fresh parsley and ¹/₂ teaspoon dried cilantro (coriander
 leaf)

Place all of the ingredients, except the cilantro, in a food processor fitted with a metal blade and blend until smooth and creamy.

Stir in the cilantro. Let the dip rest one hour to release all the flavor. Adjust any of the ingredients to your taste. Whip with a spoon before serving.

SERVES 8
1 tablespoon per serving

	Fat (g)	Cholesterol (g)	Sodium (mg)	Calories
Total Recipe	64	0	136	768
Per Portion	8	0	17	96

Hommos

Hommos makes a great dip with pita bread triangles or a spread for a pita bread pocket sandwich with shredded lettuce and tomato. The chickpeas or garbanzo beans are high in fiber. Tahini can be purchased in most supermarkets and gourmet markets.

2 cups cooked garbanzo beans
¹/₄ cup plus 1 tablespoon tahini (sesame seed paste)
¹/₂ cup fresh lemon juice (juice of 3–4 lemons)
1 tablespoon extra virgin olive oil
2¹/₂ teaspoons fresh chopped garlic
2 tablespoons water
1 tablespoon chopped fresh parsley

Blend all ingredients, except the parsley, in the blender or food processor until smooth and creamy.

If the garlic is not very fresh you may need to add more. Feel free to add extra water to achieve the consistency you wish.

Let the hommos rest for at least 30 minutes before serving. Top with parsley. The recipe makes 2 cups.

SERVES 8

1/4 cup servings

	Fat (g)	Cholesterol (g)	Sodium (mg)	Calories
Total Recipe	51.2	0	1448	1095.2
Per Portion	6.4	0	181	136.9

—— Herbed Ricotta Cheese ——

Low in calories and fat and high in flavor, this cheese can be used in pocket sandwiches, on pizzas, and as a spread for toasted crusty bread or crackers. By opting to leave out the salt you can reduce your sodium by 125 milligrams per serving.

1 pint ricotta cheese (any with at least 1/3 less fat than regular part-skim ricotta)

2 tablespoons fresh rosemary leaves, chopped (or 11/2 tablespoons dried rosemary soaked in 2 tablespoons hot water to rehydrate)

2 teaspoons minced fresh garlic

1 teaspoon freshly ground black pepper

1/2 teaspoon salt, optional

Place a double layer of fine-mesh cotton cheesecloth in a large rust-proof sieve or colander. Place the sieve over a bowl large enough to collect 1 cup of whey. Place cheese on top of the cheesecloth. Cover the sieve and let rest in the refrigerator for 4–6 hours, allowing the whey to drain from the cheese.

If using rehydrated rosemary, drain the herb once it has softened. In a small bowl, mix the drained ricotta with the remaining ingredients.

SERVES 8 (1/4 cup servings)

	Fat (g)	Cholesterol (g)	Sodium (mg)	Calories
Total Recipe	40	152	1776	712
Per Portion	5	19	222	89

Pineapple and Ham Ginger Biscuits

These are a variation on the more traditional and salty ham biscuits. They are lower in sodium, fat, and calories. They can be served wherever ham biscuits are welcome: for breakfast, at a picnic, for lunch with a soup or salad, or even on a buffet table.

**2 pieces imported, extra lean ham, rinsed under cold water
    and cut into 6 pieces each
6 slices pineapple, fresh or canned
1 recipe Gingered Rolls (page 225)
1/4 teaspoon mace**

On a nonstick baking sheet, line up the 12 pieces of ham and top with a 1/2-inch slice of pineapple. Broil them 2 inches from the element for 3–4 minutes or until the ham starts to turn brown on the edges.

Sprinkle the mace over the pineapple.

Slice the rolls and fill each one with a ham and pineapple package. The recipe makes 12 biscuits.

SERVES 6
2 biscuits per serving

	Fat (g)	Cholesterol (g)	Sodium (mg)	Calories
Total Recipe	22.8	0	852	2179.8
Per Portion	3.8	0	142	363.3

— Focaccia Sandwich with — Asparagus and Lemon Tarragon Sauce

This is a light and refreshing sandwich. It's always satisfying to bite down into a sandwich, and it's even better when it's good for you. If you don't have any homemade (and lower fat) Focaccia on hand, this bread can be found in some gourmet stores.

½ loaf of Focaccia with Fresh Sage (page 224)
2 vine-ripened tomatoes or 4 plum tomatoes
4 tablespoons Lemon Tarragon Dressing (page 170)
¼ cucumber, peeled
½ pound asparagus, steamed until tender and chilled

Use freshly baked bread for tenderness. Slice the bread into four wedges and slice each through the middle to form two sandwich slices.

Slice the tomatoes and cucumber wafer-thin.

Layer the tomatoes, asparagus, and cucumber on the bread and top with a tablespoon of sauce.

SERVES 4

	Fat (g)	Cholesterol (g)	Sodium (mg)	Calories
Total Recipe	14.8	.4	111.2	990.8
Per Portion	3.7	.1	27.8	247.7

Focaccia with Slaw and Swiss Cheese

This sandwich has the appeal of a big sandwich with melted cheese. If you use low-sodium Dijon mustard, you can lower the sodium content by 57 milligrams per serving.

1/2 loaf Focaccia with Fresh Sage (page 224)
4 servings of Caraway Slaw (page 119)
2 ounces sliced low-sodium Swiss cheese (8 milligrams sodium/ounce)
2 teaspoons Dijon mustard

Use only fresh bread for tenderness. Slice the bread into 4 wedges and slice them through the center to form two sandwich slices apiece.

Spread the mustard on one side of the bread; top with the slaw and then the cheese.

Place both halves under the broiler 2 inches from the element until the cheese starts to bubble and the bread turns golden brown.

Serve warm.

SERVES 4

	Fat (g)	Cholesterol (g)	Sodium (mg)	Calories
Total Recipe	36	0	636	1290.8
Per Portion	9	0	159	322.7

▪ *Appendices* ▪

APPENDIX 1

Calorie, Fat, and Cholesterol
Content of Commonly Used Foods

Caloric Value (Kcal), Fat, and
Cholesterol Content of Commonly
Used Foods*

Food	Amounts	Kcal	Fat (gm)	Cholesterol (mg)
APPLE				
Raw	1 medium	70	trace (tr)	0
Baked, with sugar	1 medium	120	tr	13
Brown Betty	1/2 cup	175	4	20
Juice or cider	1/2 cup	60	tr	0
Pie (see PIES)				
Applesauce, canned				
sweetened	1/2 cup	115	tr	0
canned unsweetened	1/2 cup	50	tr	0
APRICOT				
Fresh	3 small	55	tr	0
Canned in syrup	1/2 cup or 4 medium halves	110	tr	0
Dried, stewed with sugar	1/2 cup or 8 medium halves	135	tr	0
Nectar	1/2 cup	70	tr	0
ASPARAGUS, cooked	1/2 cup	15	tr	0
AVOCADO, raw	1/2 medium	185	19	0
BACON				
Broiled or fried	2 slices, cooked crisp	90	8	14
Canadian, cooked	3 slices, cooked crisp (1.5 ozs.)	100	12	20
BANANA, raw	1 medium, 6 inches long	100	tr	0
BEANS				
Sprouts, mung, cooked	1/2 cup	18		
raw	1 cup	25	tr	0
Green snap, cooked	1/2 cup	15	tr	0
Green lima, cooked	1/2 cup	130	tr	0

* Data from B.K. Watt and A.L. Merrill, *Composition of Foods—Raw, Processed and Prepared*, U.S. Department of Agriculture, Washington, D.C., 1963; *Nutritive Value of Foods*, Home and Garden Bulletin no. 72, rev., U.S. Department of Agriculture, Washington, D.C., 1971.

Food	Amounts	Kcal	Fat (gm)	Cholesterol (mg)
Baby green lima, cooked	1/2 cup	100	tr	0
Red kidney, canned	1/2 cup	115	1	0
White, canned with tomato sauce, without pork	1/2 cup	155	3	0
White, canned with tomato sauce, with pork	1/2 cup	155	3	3
Lentils (see LENTILS)				
BEEF				
Corned, canned	3 ounces	185	10	56
Corned hash, canned	1/2 cup	155	10	23
Dried or chipped	2 ounces (4 thin slices)	115	4	38
Ground, broiled	3 ounces (1 patty, 3 inch diameter)	245	17	60
Heart, braised	3 ounces	160	5	235
Liver, fried	2 ounces	130	6	250
Meat loaf, baked	1 slice	240	17	45
Potpie	1 pie, 41/2-inch diameter	560	33	41
Pot roast, cooked	3 ounces	245	16	70
Roast, cooked	3 ounces	165	7	60
Steak, lean (sirloin), broiled	3 ounces	178	9	77
Steak, regular (rib eye), broiled	3 ounces	330	30	80
Stroganoff, cooked	1/2 cup	250	18	65
Stew	1 cup	245	11	72
Tongue, braised	3 ounces	210	14	120
BEETS, cooked	1/2 cup	28	tr	0
BEVERAGES				
Carbonated, soft drinks	12 ounces (1 can)	150	0	0
Club soda	12 ounces	0	0	0
Ginger ale	12 ounces (1 can)	110	0	0
BISCUITS, baking powder	1 biscuit, 2-inch diameter	105	5	2
BLACKBERRIES, raw	1/2 cup	45	1	0
BLUEBERRIES, raw	1/2 cup	45	1	0
BOLOGNA, beef	2 ounces (2 slices)	146	13	26
BOUILLON CUBES	1 cube	5	tr	0
BREAD				
Boston brown	1 slice, 3 × 3/4 inch	100	1	1
Cracked wheat	1 slice	65	1	1
French or Vienna	1 slice, 3 inches	60	1	0
Italian	1 slice, 3 inches	55	tr	1
Light or dark rye	1 slice	60	tr	1
Pumpernickel	1 slice	85	1	1
Raisin	1 slice	65	1	1
White	1 slice	70	1	1
Whole wheat	1 slice	60	1	1

Food	Amounts	Kcal	Fat (gm)	Cholesterol (mg)
Crumbs	1/4 cup	98	1	1
BROCCOLI, cooked	1/2 cup	20	1	0
raw	1 cup	20	1	0
BRUSSELS SPROUTS,				
cooked	1/2 cup (5 medium)	28	1	0
BUNS (see ROLLS)				
BUTTER	1 tablespoon	100	12	31
CABBAGE				
Cooked	1/2 cup	15	tr	0
Raw	1/2 cup	10	tr	0
CAKE				
Angel food, without icing	1 slice (12 slices/cake)	135	tr	0
Boston cream pie	1 slice (12 slices/cake)	210	6	53
Coffee cake, with icing	1 slice, 3 × 3 × 1 1/4 inches	260	11	30
Plain cupcakes, with icing	1	130	5	54
Plain cupcakes, without				
icing	1	90	3	47
Chocolate cake, 2 layer,				
with chocolate or				
vanilla icing	1 slice (16 slices/cake)	235	9	29
Fruitcake	1 slice (30 slices/loaf)	55	2	7
Pound, without icing	1 slice (1 ounce)	140	9	30
Sponge, without icing	1 slice (12 slices/cake)	195	4	162
White cake, 2 layer, with				
chocolate or vanilla				
icing	1 slice (16 slices/cake)	250	8	31
CANDY				
Caramels	4 small	115	3	2
Plain chocolate	1 ounce	150	9	3
Chocolate with almonds	1.8 ounces	265	19	7
Chocolate creams	1 ounce (2 pieces)	110	4	4
Chocolate fudge	1 ounce (1 inch square)	115	4	5
Hard	1 ounce (6 pieces)	110	tr	0
Peanut brittle	1 ounce (1 piece)	124	4	2
CANTALOUPE	1/2 melon	60	tr	0
CARROTS				
raw	1 or 1/2 cup grated	20	tr	0
cooked	1/2 cup	23	tr	0
CATSUP, Tomato	1 tablespoon	18	tr	0
CAULIFLOWER, cooked	1/2 cup	13	tr	0
raw	1 cup	13	tr	0
CELERY, raw	1 stalk or 1/2 cup	18	tr	0
cooked	1 cup	16	tr	0
CEREALS				
Bran flakes, 40% bran	1 ounce (3/4 cup)	80	1	0
Cooked, all types	2/3 cup	87	1	0
Corn flakes	1 ounce (1 1/3 cup)	130	tr	0
Puffed rice	1 ounce (2 cups)	120	tr	0

Food	Amounts	Kcal	Fat (gm)	Cholesterol (mg)
Rice flakes	1 ounce (1 cup)	115	tr	0
Wheat flakes	1 ounce (1 cup)	105	tr	0
Shredded Wheat	1 ounce (1 biscuit or 1/2 cup)	90	1	0
CHEESE				
Blue (Roquefort type)	1 ounce	105	9	21
Brie	1 ounce	95	8	28
Cheddar (American)	1 ounce	115	10	30
Cheddar (American), grated	1 tablespoon	30	2	8
Cottage, creamed (4% fat)	1/2 cup	120	5	17
Cottage, low-fat (2% fat)	1/2 cup	100	2	8
Cream	1 tablespoon	45	6	17
Mozzarella, part-skim	1 ounce	80	5	16
Swiss (domestic)	1 ounce	105	8	35
Sauce	1/4 cup	110	9	43
Souffle	3/4 cup	200	16	132
CHEESECAKE	1 slice (10 slices/cake)	400	23	114
CHERRIES, raw sweet	1 cup	80	tr	0
CHICKPEAS, dry raw (garbanzos)	1/2 cup	380	5	0
CHICKEN				
Broiled or baked	3 ounces, without bone or skin	115	2	66
Canned	3 ounces (1/3 cup) deboned	170	10	77
Creamed	1/2 cup	222	12	93
Breast, fried	3 ounces (1/2 breast) with bone	155	5	55
Drumstick, fried	1 with bone	90	4	43
Pot pie, baked	1 pie, 41/4 inch diameter	535	31	13
CHILI				
Con carne with beans, canned	3/4 cup	250	11	25
Con carne without beans, canned	3/4 cup	383	29	30
Sauce	1 tablespoon	20	tr	0
CHOCOLATE				
Bitter	1 ounce (1 square)	145	15	0
Candy (see CANDY)				
Flavored milk drink	1 cup (made with skim milk)	190	6	8
Morsels	30 morsels or 11/2 tablespoons	80	4	1
Syrup	2 tablespoons	80	tr	2
CHOP SUEY, cooked	3/4 cup	325	20	32
COCOA, beverage	3/4 cup (made with milk)	176	8	26

Food	Amounts	Kcal	Fat (gm)	Cholesterol (mg)
COCONUT				
Dried, shredded, sweetened	1/4 cup	85	6	0
Fresh shredded	1/4 cup	113	12	0
COLE SLAW, with cabbage	1/2 cup	50	4	4
COOKIES				
Brownies	1 piece, 2 × 2 × 1/2 inch	145	9	22
Chocolate chip	1 cookie, 2 inch diameter	60	3	6
Coconut bar chews	1 cookie, 2 inch diameter	55	2	6
Oatmeal with raisins and nuts	1 cookie, 2 inch diameter	65	4	4
Sugar, plain	1 cookie, 2 1/2 inch diameter	40	2	7
CORN				
Sweet, cooked	1 ear, 5 inches long	70	1	0
Canned	1/2 cup	85	1	0
Grits, cooked	2/3 cup	85	tr	0
Muffins	1 muffin, 2 1/2 inch diameter	125	4	2
Cornmeal, dry	1 cup, white or yellow	500	2	0
CRACKERS				
Graham, plain	2 squares	55	1	8
Saltines	2 crackers	35	1	6
CRANBERRY				
Juice	1/2 cup	85	tr	0
Sauce, canned	1/4 cup	85	tr	0
CREAM				
Light cream	1 tablespoon	30	3	10
Half-and-half	1 tablespoon	20	2	6
Heavy, whipping	1 tablespoon, unwhipped	55	6	24
CREAMER (imitation cream)	1 teaspoon powder	10	1	0
CUCUMBER, raw	1/2	5	tr	0
CUSTARD, baked	1/2 cup	143	7	133
DATES, pitted	8 or 1/4 cup	123	tr	4
DOUGHNUTS, cake-type	1	125	6	26
EGG				
Raw, boiled, or poached	1 whole egg	80	6	252
White	1 egg white	15	tr	0
Yolk	1 egg yolk	60	5	252
Fried	1 egg, cooked in 1 teaspoon fat	115	10	265
Scrambled	1 egg (milk and fat added)	110	8	267
Eggnog	1/2 cup	335	19	73
ENDIVE, curly, raw	1/2 cup	10	tr	0
FARINA, cooked	2/3 cup	70	tr	0
FATS				
Cooking, lard	1 tablespoon	115	13	12
Cooking, vegetable	1 tablespoon	110	13	0

Food	Amounts	Kcal	Fat (gm)	Cholesterol (mg)
FIGS				
Dried	1 large	60	tr	0
Fresh, raw	3 small	90	tr	0
FISH				
Bluefish, baked	3 ounces	135	4	60
Codfish (dried)	1/2 cup	190	2	42
Clams, raw	3 ounces	65	1	42
Clams, canned	1/2 cup (3 medium)	80	2	50
Crab, fresh	3 ounces	80	2	85
Crab, canned	1/2 cup	100	2	85
Fish sticks, breaded, cooked	5 sticks, each 4 × 1 × 1/2 inches	200	10	80
Flounder, baked	3 ounces	85	1	59
Haddock, pan-fried	3 ounces	140	5	51
Lobster, cooked	3 ounces (1/2 cup)	90	1	70
Mackerel, baked	3 ounces	210	14	77
Oysters, raw	1/2 cup (8–10 oysters)	80	2	60
Oyster stew with milk	1 cup with 3–4 oysters	200	12	30
Perch, pan-fried	3 ounces	195	11	51
Salmon, red, cooked	3 ounces	140	5	60
Salmon, pink, canned	3 ounces (1/2 cup)	120	5	34
Salmon loaf	4 ounces (1 slice)	235	10	72
Sardines, canned in oil	3 ounces	175	7	85
Shrimp	3 ounces (1/2 cup)	100	1	115
Sole, baked	3 ounces	85	1	59
Trout, baked	3 ounces	85	1	59
Tuna, white, oil-packed	3 ounces (1/2 cup)	170	7	55
Tuna, white, water-packed	3 ounces (1/2 cup)	120	1	55
Tuna salad (see SALAD, TUNAFISH)	1/2 cup	25	18	42
FRANKFURTER	1 frankfurter	170	15	29
FRENCH TOAST, fried	1 slice	180	12	135
FRUIT COCKTAIL, canned in syrup	1/2 cup	98	tr	0
GELATIN				
Plain, dry	1 tablespoon (1 envelope)	25	tr	0
Dessert, plain, prepared	1/2 cup	70	0	0
GINGERBREAD	1 slice (2 1/2 inch square)	175	4	0
GRAPEFRUIT				
White or pink, raw	1/2 medium	45	tr	0
Canned, in syrup	1/2 cup	88	tr	0
Juice, unsweetened	1/2 cup	50	tr	0
GRAPES				
Raw	1 cup	110	tr	0
Juice	1/2 cup	83	tr	0
GREENS				
Collards, cooked	1/2 cup	28	1	0

Food	Amounts	Kcal	Fat (gm)	Cholesterol (mg)
Dandelion, cooked	1/2 cup	30	1	0
Kale, cooked	1/2 cup	15	1	0
Mustard, cooked	1/2 cup	18	1	0
Spinach, cooked	1/2 cup	20	1	0
Turnip, cooked	1/2 cup	15	tr	0
GUAVAS, raw	1	50	tr	0
HAM				
Boiled	3 ounces	200	15	77
Cured, roasted	3 ounces	245	19	77
Luncheon, deviled, canned	2 tablespoons	165	14	28
ICE CREAM				
Ice cream (10% fat)	1/2 cup	145	9	39
Ice cream, rich (16% fat)	1/2 cup	180	12	44
Ice cream, specialty (22% fat)	1/2 cup	300	23	153
ICE MILK	1/2 cup	100	4	13
JAMS, jellies, preserves	1 tablespoon	55	tr	0
LAMB				
Chop, cooked	3 ounces, without bone, fat-trimmed	185	9	80
Leg, roasted	3 ounces, without bone, fat-trimmed	160	6	75
LEMON JUICE	1 tablespoon	5	tr	0
LEMONADE, sweetened	1 cup	110	tr	0
LENTILS, all types, cooked	1/2 cup	120	tr	0
LETTUCE, all types	1 cup	10	tr	0
LIME JUICE	1/4 cup	15	tr	0
LIVER				
Beef, fried	2 ounces	130	6	250
Calf, fried	2.5 ounces	230	15	324
Chicken, fried	3 ounces (3 medium)	235	15	634
Pork, fried	2.5 ounces	225	15	307
MACARONI				
Cooked	3/4 cup	115	1	0
Macaroni and cheese, baked	3/4 cup	325	17	32
MANGOES, raw	1 medium	90	0	0
MARGARINE	1 tablespoon	100	12	0
MARSHMALLOWS	1 large	25	0	0
MILK				
Dry skim (nonfat)	1/4 cup powder	61	tr	3
Dry whole	1/4 cup powder	129	7	25
Evaporated, canned	1/2 cup, undiluted and unsweetened	173	10	39
Low-fat (2% fat)	1 cup	120	5	17
Skim or buttermilk (made with skim milk)	1 cup	90	tr	5

Food	Amounts	Kcal	Fat (gm)	Cholesterol (mg)
Whole (4% fat)	1 cup	160	9	33
Malted, plain	1½ cup	368	15	49
Milkshake, chocolate	1½ cup	420	18	37
MOLASSES				
Cane, blackstrap	1 tablespoon	45	0	0
Cane, light	1 tablespoon	50	0	0
MUFFIN, plain	1 muffin, 2¾ inch diameter	120	4	2
MUSHROOMS, canned	½ cup	20	tr	0
raw	10 small	28	0	0
NOODLES, egg, cooked	¾ cup	150	2	43
NUTS				
Almonds	¼ cup	213	19	0
Cashews, roasted	¼ cup	196	16	0
Peanuts, roasted	¼ cup	210	18	0
Pecan halves	¼ cup	185	19	0
Walnut halves	¼ cup	163	16	0
OATMEAL OR ROLLED OATS, cooked	⅔ cup	87	1	0
OILS, salad or cooking, all types	1 tablespoon	125	14	0
OKRA, cooked	4 medium	13	tr	0
OLIVES				
Green	4 medium or 3 large	15	2	0
Black	2 large	37	2	0
ONION				
raw	1 medium	40	2	0
cooked	½ cup	30	tr	0
ORANGE				
Fresh	1 medium	65	tr	0
Juice	½ cup	60	tr	0
PANCAKE, wheat or white	1 medium, 5 inch diameter	60	2	16
PAPAYAS, raw	½ cup	35	tr	0
PARSLEY, raw	1 tablespoon chopped	tr	tr	0
PARSNIPS, cooked	½ cup	50	1	0
PEACHES				
Canned in syrup	½ cup	100	tr	0
Canned in water	½ cup	40	tr	0
Fresh or frozen	1 small or ½ cup	35	tr	0
PEANUT BUTTER	2 tablespoons	190	16	0
PEARS				
Canned in syrup	2 medium halves or ½ cup	90	tr	0
Fresh	1 medium	100	1	0
PEAS				
Cowpeas or blackeyed peas, cooked	½ cup	95	1	0
Green, cooked	½ cup	58	1	0
Split, cooked	½ cup	145	1	0

Food	Amounts	Kcal	Fat (gm)	Cholesterol (mg)
PEPPER				
Green, stuffed with meat	1 medium, cooked	200	14	34
Fresh, green or red	1 medium without stem and seeds	15	tr	0
PERSIMMONS, fresh	1 fruit, 2¹/₂ inch diameter	75	tr	0
PICKLE				
Relish	1 tablespoon	20	tr	0
Dill	1 large	10	tr	0
PIE (9 inch diameter)				
Apple	1 slice (8 slices/pie)	300	13	36
Cherry	¹/₈ pie	300	13	12
Custard	¹/₈ pie	250	12	120
Lemon meringue	¹/₈ pie	270	10	97
Mince	¹/₈ pie	320	14	14
Pumpkin	¹/₈ pie	240	15	70
PINEAPPLE				
Canned in syrup	2 small slices or ¹/₂ cup	90	tr	0
Fresh	¹/₂ cup	38	tr	0
Juice, unsweetened	¹/₂ cup	68	tr	0
PIZZA (cheese)	¹/₈ of 14 inch diameter pie	185	6	31
PLANTAIN, fresh, green	1 baking banana, 6 inches long	135	0	0
PLUMS				
Canned, in syrup	¹/₂ cup or 3 small plums	100	tr	0
Raw	1 plum	25	tr	0
POPCORN, popped	1 cup (oil added)	40	2	0
PORK				
Pork chop, loin, lean	5.3 ounces, fat trimmed w/ bone before cooking	166	7.5	71
Pork chop, w/out fat trimmed	5.3 ounces w/bone before cooking	275	19.2	84
Roast loin, lean	3 ounces	204	11.9	77
POTATO				
Potato chips	10 medium	115	8	0
Baked or boiled	1 medium	90	tr	0
French fried	10 pieces	115	7	11
Mashed	¹/₂ cup (milk and butter added)	95	4	15
PRETZELS	5, 3¹/₈ inch sticks	10	tr	0
PRUNES				
Dried, cooked with sugar	5 medium	160	tr	0
Juice	¹/₂ cup	100	tr	0
PUDDING				
Chocolate blanc mange	¹/₂ cup	190	8	12
Cornstarch	¹/₂ cup	140	5	18
Rice with raisins	¹/₂ cup	300	8	15
Tapioca	¹/₂ cup	140	5	8
RADISHES, raw	4 small	5	tr	0

Food	Amounts	Kcal	Fat (gm)	Cholesterol (mg)
RAISINS, seedless	1 tablespoon	30	tr	0
RASPBERRIES, raw, red	1/2 cup	35	1	0
RHUBARB, cooked with sugar	1/2 cup	190	tr	0
RICE, cooked, all varieties	3/4 cup	140	tr	0
ROLLS				
Bagel (egg)	1 roll, 3 inch diameter	165	2	85
Barbecue bun	1 bun, 3 1/2 inch diameter	120	2	1
Hard	1 large round	160	2	1
Plain, white	1 small dinner roll	85	2	1
Cinnamon	1 roll	135	4	30
RUTABAGAS, cooked	1/2 cup	25	tr	0
SALAD				
Chicken	1/2 cup, with mayonnaise	280	19	36
Egg	1/2 cup, with mayonnaise	190	18	262
Fresh fruit	1/2 cup, with French dressing	130	6	1
Jellied, vegetable	1/2 cup, no dressing	70	0	0
Lettuce	1 cup, with French dressing	80	6	2
Potato	1/2 cup, with mayonnaise	185	12	37
Tomato aspic	1/2 cup, no dressing	45	0	0
Tuna fish	1/2 cup, with mayonnaise	250	18	42
SALAD DRESSING				
Blue cheese	1 tablespoon	75	8	9
French	1 tablespoon	65	6	16
Low-calorie, oil-free	2 tablespoons	17	0	2
Mayonnaise	1 tablespoon	100	11	10
Thousand Island	1 tablespoon	80	8	5
SAUCE				
Chocolate	2 tablespoons	75	4	2
Custard	2 tablespoons (low-calorie, with nonfat dry milk)	45	1	16
Hard	1 tablespoon	90	6	20
Hollandaise (mock)	2 tablespoons	75	7	84
Lemon	2 tablespoons	40	1	35
SAUERKRAUT, canned	1/2 cup	25	tr	0
SAUSAGE				
Liverwurst	2 ounces	150	12	198
Pork, cooked	2 small patties or links	125	11	26
Vienna	1 canned, 2 inches long	40	3	11
SHERBET, orange	1/2 cup	130	1	7
SYRUP, table blends	1 tablespoon, light and dark	60	0	0
SOUP				
Bean with pork, canned	1 cup	170	6	10
Beef broth, bouillon, consomme, canned	1 cup	30	0	0
Chicken noodle, canned	1 cup	65	2	6

Food	Amounts	Kcal	Fat (gm)	Cholesterol (mg)
Clam chowder, canned	1 cup	85	3	38
Cream of vegetable (e.g., tomato, mushroom), canned	1 cup	135	10	31
Gumbo	1 cup	140	1	0
Lentil	1 cup	140	1	0
Minestrone, canned	1 cup	105	3	2
Tomato, canned	1 cup	90	3	5
Vegetable, canned	1 cup	80	2	0
SPAGHETTI				
Cooked	3/4 cup	115	1	0
In tomato sauce, with meat balls	3/4 cup	250	9	56
SPINACH (see GREENS)				
SQUASH, summer, cooked	1/2 cup	15	tr	0
STRAWBERRIES, raw	1/2 cup	30	1	0
SUGAR				
Brown	1 tablespoon	50	0	0
Granulated	1 tablespoon	40	0	0
Lump	1 cube	25	0	0
Powdered	1 tablespoon	30	0	0
SWEET POTATO				
Baked	1 medium	155	1	0
Candied	1 medium	295	6	0
TANGERINE	1 medium	40	tr	0
TARTAR SAUCE (see SALAD DRESSING, Mayonnaise)				
TOAST, melba	1 slice	20	tr	0
TOMATO				
Ketchup	1 tablespoon	15	tr	0
Juice, canned	1/2 cup	23	tr	0
Canned	1/2 cup	25	1	0
Raw	1 medium	40	4	0
TOPPING, whipped	1 tablespoon	10	1	3
TORTILLAS	1 tortilla, 5-inch diameter	50	1	0
TURKEY				
with skin	3 ounces	180	8	70
without skin	3 ounces	150	4	65
TURNIP				
Greens (see GREENS)				
Cooked	1/2 cup	18	tr	0
VEAL				
Cutlet, breaded (wiener schnitzel)	4.8 ounces	315	21	122
Cutlet, lean	3 ounces before trimming	140	3.5	106.2
Roast, lean	3 ounces before trimming	123	4.3	104.7
VINEGAR	1 tablespoon	2	0	0
WAFFLES	1 waffle, 7 inch diameter	210	7	54

Food	Amounts	Kcal	Fat (gm)	Cholesterol (mg)
WATERMELON, raw	1 wedge or 1 cup	115	1	0
WELSH RAREBIT	½ cup	330	26	114
WHEAT FLOUR				
White	1 cup	420	1	0
Whole wheat	1 cup	400	2	0
Wheat germ	2 tablespoons	30	1	0
WHITE SAUCE	¼ cup	110	8	8
YEAST				
Brewers, dry	1 tablespoon	25	tr	0
Compressed	1 ounce cake	25	tr	0
Dry active	4 packages (1 ounce each)	80	tr	0
YOGURT, plain, low-fat	1 cup	125	4	15

APPENDIX 2

Low-Cholesterol, Low-Saturated Fat Diet I

Approximate Composition:
    Calories: 1655   Protein: 78 gm
    Fat: 35 gm   Carbohydrate: 257 gm

FOOD	TO INCLUDE	TO AVOID
BEVERAGE	Tea, coffee, cocoa made with skim milk, carbonated beverages	All other
BREAD	All, except hot breads	Hot breads, unless made with fat allowance
CEREAL	All	None
CHEESE	Cottage cheese, ricotta, and other cheeses made totally from skim milk	All other
DESSERT	Fruit ice, jello, fruit whips made with egg white, puddings made with skim milk, angel food and plain white cake, vanilla wafers	Pies, pastries, rich cakes, cookies, ice cream, pudding made with whole milk and/or egg yolk
EGG	One egg daily, if desired* (egg whites, as desired)	Fried eggs or others prepared with fat
FAT	Small amounts of butter, fortified margarine, or salad oil, if desired	Gravies, cream, cream sauces, nuts, peanut butter, olives, chocolate

FOOD	TO INCLUDE	TO AVOID
FRUIT	Fruit and fruit juices, as tolerated	Avocado; the following may not be well tolerated: apples, melons
MEAT, FISH, FOWL	Five ounces daily: *lean* beef, lamb, pork, veal, chicken, turkey, fish	All fatty meat, all fried meat, duck, goose, fatty fish, luncheon meat, dried or smoked meat or fish, fish in oil
MILK	3 cups skim milk or skim buttermilk, skim milk yogurt	All other
POTATO OR SUBSTITUTE	Potato, rice, noodles, macaroni, spaghetti	All fried and creamed, potato chips
SOUP	Fat free broth or consomme, other soups made with allowed foods	All other
SWEETS	Sugar, jelly, molasses, syrup, honey, hard candy	Chocolate
VEGETABLE	All, as tolerated	The following may not be well tolerated: broccoli, brussels sprouts, cauliflower, cabbage, corn, cucumber, radishes, onions, peppers, turnips, lima beans, dried peas and beans
MISCELLANEOUS	Spices and condiments as tolerated	All other

*When egg is not taken, one ounce of *lean* meat may be added.
For a minimum-fat diet (20 grams): Omit butter, margarine, salad oil; use egg only as meat substitute.

SUGGESTED MEAL PATTERN

BREAKFAST		
	Fruit or juice	1/2 cup
	Cereal	1/2 cup
	Egg	1
	Bread	1 slice
	Butter or fortified margarine	1 tsp.
	Jelly	1 Tbsp.
	Sugar	3 tsp.
	Milk, skim	1 cup
	Beverage	

LUNCH	Juice	1/2 cup
	Meat or substitute	2 ounces
	Potato or substitute	1/2 cup
	Vegetable	1/2 cup
	Bread	1 slice
	Jelly	1 Tbsp.
	Fruit	1/2 cup
	Milk, skim	1 cup
	Sugar	2 tsp.
	Beverage	
DINNER	Juice	1/2 cup
	Meat or substitute	3 ounces
	Potato or substitute	1/2 cup
	Vegetable	1/2 cup
	Salad, fruit	1/2 cup
	Bread	1 slice
	Jelly	1 Tbsp.
	Dessert	1/2 cup
	Milk, skim	1 cup
	Sugar	2 tsp.

Low-Cholesterol, Low-Saturated Fat Diet II

This is a fat-controlled diet in which the amount and type of fat are carefully regulated. About 30% of the day's calories will come from fat. More of the fat will be the polyunsaturated (vegetable oil) rather than the saturated (meat and dairy products).

Approximate Composition:
Calories: 1800   Protein: 67 gm
Fat: 60 gm   Carbohydrate: 248 gm
Cholesterol: 225 mg
Sat. Fatty Acids: 9.5 gm

FOOD	TO INCLUDE	TO AVOID
BEVERAGE (non-dairy)	Coffee, tea, carbonated beverages, cocoa made with skim milk	Hot chocolate
BREAD	Whole grain biscuits, muffins; griddle cakes and cornbread must be home made with an allowed fat or oil, containing no whole milk or egg yolk. The amount served must be counted as part of the daily fat allowance	Commercial biscuits, muffins, griddle cakes, cornbread, coffee cakes, crackers, mixes for biscuits, muffins, doughnuts, sweet rolls

FOOD	TO INCLUDE	TO AVOID
CEREAL	All	None
CHEESE	Cottage, ricotta, and any cheese made with skim milk	Cream cheese, hard cheese, or any other made with whole milk
DESSERT	Tapioca, cornstarch pudding made with skim milk, fruit whip, gelatin, fruit ice, fruit, angel food cake, skim-milk yogurt desserts, cornflake and nut meringues, homemade desserts if all ingredients are allowed	Puddings, custard and ice cream unless made with skim milk or nonfat dry milk powder, whipped cream desserts, pies, cakes, and cookies unless homemade with allowed fat or oil
EGG	Not more than three per week used plain or in cooking. Use egg white as desired	Foods made with egg yolk (i.e. egg noodles) unless counted as part of allowance
FAT	5 servings unsaturated fats such as oil (corn, cottonseed, safflower, sesame seed, soybean, sunflower seed), margarine made from these oils, mayonnaise, french dressing with allowed oil	Butter, hydrogenated margarines and shortenings, lard, salt pork, chicken fat, coconut oil, palm oil, olive oil, peanut oil
FRUIT	All, one of which should be a source of Vitamin C daily. Emphasize raw fruit. Avocado may be used in small amounts.	None
MEAT, FISH FOWL	*Leaner:* veal, chicken, turkey (remove all visible fat) 4–5 times a week. *Fattier:* beef, lamb (leg roast), pork and ham (remove all visible fat) 3–4 times per week. *Fish:* in unrestricted amounts; shellfish total 5 oz. daily, including shrimp. Latest research indicates that cholesterol content of shellfish, including shrimp, is comparable to that found in chicken, lean	Fatty cuts of beef, lamb or pork, bacon, salt pork and spare ribs, frankfurters, sausage, cold cuts, canned meats; organ meats (kidney, brain, sweetbreads, liver, and gizzards) any visible fat from meat, goose, the skin of chicken or turkey, fish canned in olive oil

FOOD	TO INCLUDE	TO AVOID
	beef and fin fish—approx. 100 mg. per 3.5 oz. serving.	
MILK	1 pint daily: fat-free skim milk, nonfat dry milk powder, buttermilk made from skim milk, evaporated skim milk or yogurt made from skim milk, polyunsaturated non-dairy creamers	Whole milk and whole milk products, homogenized milk, sweet and powdered cream, ice cream unless homemade with nonfat dry milk powder, sour cream, butter milk or yogurt made from whole milk, non-dairy creamers made with saturated fat
POTATO OR SUBSTITUTE	All, except fried	All fried potato products, potato chips
SOUP	Fat free: consommé, bouillon, vegetable soup, or cream soup made with skim milk	Cream soup made with whole milk
SWEETS	Sugar, jam, jelly, syrup, etc.	Chocolate, candies made with chocolate, butter or cream
VEGETABLE	All. Include a source of vitamin A four times weekly. Emphasize raw vegetables	None
MISCELLANEOUS	Pickles, relishes, vinegar, mustard, ketchup and seasonings, nuts except those excluded	Sauces and gravies unless made with allowed fat or oil or made from skimmed stock, frozen or packaged dinners, olives, coconut, cashew or macadamia nuts, commercial popcorn, Fritos, cheese puffs, etc.

Suggested Meal Pattern

BREAKFAST	Fruit or juice	1/2 cup
	Cereal	1/2 cup
	Egg (3 per week)	
	Fortified margarine	1 tsp.
	Bread	1 slice
	Jelly	1 Tbsp.
	Sugar	3 tsp.
	Milk, skim	1 cup
	Beverage	

LUNCH	Fat-free soup	1 cup
	Lean meat or substitute	3 ounces
	Potato or substitute	1/2 cup
	Vegetable	1/2 cup
	Salad, vegetable	3/4 cup
	Salad oil	1 tsp.
	Bread	1 slice
	Fortified margarine	1 tsp.
	Fruit	1/2 cup
	Milk, skim	1/2 cup
	Sugar	2 tsp.
	Beverage	
DINNER	Juice	1/2 cup
	Lean meat or substitute	3 ounces
	Potato or substitute	1/2 cup
	Vegetable	1/2 cup
	Salad, vegetable	3/4 cup
	Salad oil	1 tsp.
	Bread	1 slice
	Fortified margarine	1 tsp.
	Jelly	1 Tbsp.
	Dessert	1/2 cup
	Sugar	2 tsp.
	Beverage	

APPENDIX 3

Sodium Content of Common Foods

Food	Serving Size	Sodium (mg)
MEATS, FISH, AND POULTRY		
bacon, Canadian	3-ounce slice	537
bacon, regular	2 thick slices	245
beef, lean	3 ounces	55
corned beef	3 ounces	802
ham, cured	3 ounces	795
lamb	3 ounces	58
pork, fresh, lean	3 ounces	59
sirloin steak, broiled	3 ounces	67
veal	3 ounces	69
halibut, broiled with butter	3 ounces	114
herring, smoked	3 ounces	5,234
shrimp, raw	3 ounces	120
shrimp, canned	3 ounces	1,955

Food	Serving Size	Sodium (mg)
chicken, dark meat	4 ounces	100
chicken, drumstick with skin	1 drumstick	47
chicken, white meat	4 ounces	75
turkey, white meat	4 ounces	93
PROCESSED MEATS		
bologna	1 slice	260
frankfurter	1 frank	627
salami, beef	1 slice	255
PREPARED DISHES		
cheeseburger	1 burger	709
hamburger	1 burger	461
pizza, with cheese (14 inch)	1/8 pie	456
pizza, with sausage (14 inch)	1/8 pie	488
chicken pot pie frozen	1 pie	933
PREPARED MEALS		
beef dinner, frozen	1 dinner	736
chicken dinner, fast food	1 dinner	2,243
fish dinner, frozen	1 dinner	1,011
turkey dinner, frozen	1 dinner	1,360
SOUPS		
chicken noodle soup, canned	1 cup	1,020
chicken noodle soup, low-sodium	1 cup	100
chunky beef and vegetable soup, low-sodium	1 cup	75
cream of mushroom soup, canned	1 cup	1,031
tomato soup, low-sodium	1 cup	29
vegetable beef soup, low-sodium	1 cup	51
VEGETABLES		
artichoke, cooked	1 medium	36
asparagus, cooked	1 spear	1
beans, green, cooked	1 cup	5
beets, cooked	1 cup	73
broccoli, raw	1 stalk	23
broccoli, cooked	1 stalk	18
brussels sprouts, cooked	1 medium	2
cabbage, cooked	1 cup	20
carrots, raw	1 carrot	34
carrots, cooked	1 cup	51
cauliflower, raw	1 cup	13

Food	Serving Size	Sodium (mg)
celery, raw	1 stalk	30
corn, cooked	1 ear	trace
cucumber	7 slices	2
eggplant, cooked	1 cup	2
green peppers, raw	1 large	13
kale, cooked	1 cup	47
lettuce	1 cup	5
lima beans, cooked	1 cup	2
mushrooms	1 cup	11
okra, cooked	10 pods	2
onions, dry	1 medium	10
peas, green, canned	1 cup	401
peas, green, fresh cooked	1 cup	2
potatoes, baked or broiled	1 potato	5
potatoes au gratin with cheese	1 cup	1,095
pumpkin, canned	1 cup	5
radish	4 small	2
rutabaga, cooked	1 cup	7
spinach, fresh	1 cup	39
spinach, cooked	1 cup	90
squash, summer, cooked	1 cup	2
squash, winter, baked	1 cup	2
sweet potatoes, baked or broiled	1 potato	15
tomato, raw	1 tomato	4
tomato, cooked	1 cup	10
tomato, canned	1 cup	313
tossed green salad	3 ounces	3
turnips, raw	1 cup	64
turnips, cooked	1 cup	53
FRUITS		
fruits, fresh generally	1 cup	1 to 4
cantaloupe	1/2 medium	33
fruit cup, fresh	1 cup	2
raisins	1 cup	39
BREADS		
biscuits, regular	1 biscuit	175
bread, raisin	1 slice	95
bread, rye	1 slice	139
bread, whole wheat	1 slice	132
bread, whole wheat, low-sodium	1 slice	7
bread, white	1 slice	142
bread, white, low-sodium	1 slice	7
soda crackers	2 crackers	72
crackers, low-sodium	1 cracker	1
crackers, unsalted tops (saltines)	2 crackers	50

Food	Serving Size	Sodium (mg)
Parker House rolls	1 roll	275
pretzel goldfish	10 "fish"	195
graham crackers	2 crackers	94
Ritz crackers	3 crackers	97
matzoh	1 piece	trace
melba toast, unsalted	1 slice	1
CEREALS		
corn flakes	1 ounce	256
corn flakes, low-sodium	1¼ cup	10
cream of wheat	¾ cup	2
oatmeal, regular, cooked without salt	1 cup	2
puffed rice	1 cup	1
puffed wheat	1 cup	1
shredded wheat	1 biscuit	1
CEREAL PRODUCTS		
macaroni	1 cup	1
rice, brown	1 cup	10
rice, white	1 cup	6
spaghetti	1 cup	1
DAIRY PRODUCTS		
butter, regular	1 tablespoon	140
butter, unsalted	1 tablespoon	2
buttermilk, cultured	1 cup	319
buttermilk, unsalted	1 cup	122
cheese, American	1 ounce	406
cheese, American, low-sodium	1 ounce	2
cheese, Cheddar	1 ounce	198
cheese, Cheddar, low-sodium	1 ounce	6
cheese, cottage, regular	4 ounces	260
cheese, cottage, unsalted	4 ounces	14
cheese, cottage, low-fat	4 ounces	260
cheese, Muenster	1 ounce	204
cheese, Parmesan, grated	1 ounce	247
cheese, Swiss, natural	1 ounce	201
cheese, Swiss, pasteurized processed	1 ounce	331
eggs, fresh	1 medium	54
cream	1 tablespoon	6
cream, whipping	1 tablespoon	5
margarine	1 tablespoon	140
margarine, unsalted	1 tablespoon	1
milk, whole or skim	1 cup	122
milk, low-fat	1 cup	150
milk, low-sodium	1 cup	6
milk, canned, condensed	1 cup	343
yogurt, plain	8 ounces	106

Food	Serving Size	Sodium (mg)
BEVERAGES		
beer	12 ounces	25
dessert wine	3 1/2 ounces	4
gin, rum, vodka, whiskey	1 1/2 ounces	trace
table wine	3 1/2 ounces	5
vermouth	4 ounces	4
coffee	1 cup	2
cola, regular	8 ounces	1
cola, low-calorie	8 ounces	40
fruit juice (orange, grapefruit, apple)	6 ounces	1
pineapple-and-grapefruit drink	8 ounces	80
tea	1 cup	2
CONDIMENTS		
A-1 sauce	1 tablespoon	275
barbecue sauce	1 tablespoon	130
blue cheese dressing	1 tablespoon	164
ketchup	1 tablespoon	156
ketchup, low-sodium	1 tablespoon	3
French dressing	1 tablespoon	214
French dressing, low-sodium	1 tablespoon	3
mayonnaise	1 tablespoon	89
mayonnaise, low-sodium	1 tablespoon	2
mustard	1 teaspoon	65
Russian dressing	1 tablespoon	138
soy sauce	1 tablespoon	1,319
sweetener	1 packet	5
teriyaki sauce	1 tablespoon	690
tomato sauce, low-sodium	1 tablespoon	50
tomato sauce, regular	1/2 cup	656
vinegar	1 tablespoon	trace
Worcestershire sauce	1 tablespoon	206
COOKING AIDS		
baking powder	1 teaspoon	339
baking powder, low-sodium	1 teaspoon	trace
baking soda	1 teaspoon	821
flour	1 cup	3
garlic salt	1 tablespoon	1,850
meat tenderizer	1 teaspoon	1,750
monosodium glutamate (MSG)	1 tablespoon	492
salt	1 teaspoon	2,132
sugar	1 tablespoon	trace
sugar, brown, packed	1 tablespoon	4
SNACKS		
almonds, unsalted, whole	1 cup	5
pickles, dill	1 pickle	928
pickles, dill, low-sodium	1 pickle	5

Food	Serving Size	Sodium (mg)
peanuts, dry-roasted, salted	1 cup	602
peanuts, dry-roasted, unsalted	1 cup	8
peanut butter, regular	1 tablespoon	97
peanut butter, low-sodium	1 tablespoon	1
potato chips	1 large chip	20
pretzels	1 pretzel	101

DESSERTS

chocolate chip cookies	2 cookies	69
chocolate pudding, instant	1/2 cup	161
ginger snaps	4 cookies	161
ice cream, chocolate	1 cup	153
ice cream, French vanilla	1 cup	153
ice cream, vanilla	1 cup	75
milkshake	1 shake	285
pecan pie	1/8 pie	228
tapioca pudding	1/2 cup	130

DIGESTIVE AIDS

Alka-Seltzer	1 tablet	521
Bromo-Seltzer	1 tablet	717
Rolaids	1 tablet	53

OTHER MEDICATIONS

aspirin	2 tablets	49
laxative	1 dose	250
toothpaste	1 brush	trace

APPENDIX 4

Low-Sodium Diets

These diets eliminate sodium products in the preparation and serving of food as well as restrict food high in sodium. The 500-milligram low-sodium diet is used as the basic diet for all sodium-restricted diets. The basic diet contains one (1) egg, four (4) ounces of meat, sixteen (16) ounces of milk, and no cheese. Modifications of sodium content either for the 500-milligram, 1-gram, or 2-gram sodium restrictions may be made by use of the following list.

All figures are approximate.

Food	Amount	Sodium (mg)
Powdered low-sodium milk	100 cc.	2.5
Skim milk	1 cup	150
Whole milk	1 cup	120

Food	Amount	Sodium (mg)
Dialyzed milk	100 cc.	3.5
Regular cottage cheese	1/2 cup	240
Natural hard cheese	1 ounce	200
Ice cream	1/2 cup	50
Egg	1 large	60
Meat, poultry, fresh fish	3 ounces	70
Tomato juice, regular	1/2 cup	250
White bread	1 slice	140
Cereal, dry, except All Bran	1 ounce	300
All Bran	1 ounce	500
Butter, regular	1 tsp.	45
Margarine, regular	1 tsp.	45
Cake, plain (sponge or angel)	2 ounces	65
Cake, white or yellow	2 ounces	150
Cake, devil's food	2 ounces	200
Gelatin dessert (regular flavored)	1/2 cup	50
Salt	1/4 tsp. scant	500

* Vegetables listed TO AVOID (except sauerkraut) may be used in 1/2-cup amounts which will yield approximately 25 mg. additional sodium.

500-Milligram Sodium Diet*
(Approximately 22 mg of Sodium)
(Severe Sodium Restriction)

Approximate Composition:
Calories: 1,850   Protein: 72 gm.
Fat: 63 gm.   Carbohydrate: 246 gm.

FOOD	TO INCLUDE	TO AVOID
BEVERAGE	Coffee, tea, cocoa, cereal beverage, carbonated beverages as allowed by physician. (For sodium content of specific beverages, see appendix 3)	Prepared beverage mixes, instant cocoa mixes, Dutch process cocoa, malted milk, fountain beverages
BREAD	Unsalted bread and crackers	Bread or crackers made with baking powder, baking soda, or salt
CEREAL	Enriched unsalted cooked cereal, puffed rice, puffed wheat, shredded wheat, or	Instant cooked and prepared cereals which contain salt or sodium

FOOD	TO INCLUDE	TO AVOID
	any prepared cereal without salt or sodium	
CHEESE	1/4 cup unsalted cottage cheese or 1 ounce of other unsalted cheese (to be used in place of 1 ounce of meat or other substitutions as listed on chart)	All other
**DESSERT	Unsalted custard and ice cream made from milk allowance; fruit ices; gelatin desserts without salt or sodium	Commercial sodium-containing gelatin desserts; desserts prepared with salt, baking powder, baking soda or egg white; pudding or cake mixes
EGG	One daily, if desired	None
FAT	Unsalted butter or fortified margarine; unsalted commercial or home prepared salad dressing; mayonnaise	Salted butter or margarine; bacon fat; commercial salad dressing prepared with salt or sodium
FRUIT	All fresh, canned or frozen fruit and fruit juices, one of which is a source of vitamin C	Dried or canned fruit containing a sodium preservative
MEAT, FISH, FOWL	Limit to 4 ounces daily, all prepared without salt. Fresh fish or fish canned without salt, only; liver no more than once in two weeks	Brains or kidneys; canned, salted or smoked meat or fish; frozen fish; shellfish, except oyster
MILK	1 pint daily, including that used in cooking	All other
POTATO OR SUBSTITUTE	White or sweet potatoes, rice, corn, noodles, macaroni, dried peas, and lima beans	Salted potato chips, instant potatoes
SOUP	Soup made from allowed foods	Canned, frozen, and dehydrated soup made with salt; bouillon in all forms
SWEETS	Sugar, honey, jellies, jams without sodium preservatives, homemade	Commercial candies and syrups, molasses, black licorice

FOOD	TO INCLUDE	TO AVOID
	candy from allowed foods, plain chocolate candy bars in place of 1/2 cup milk	
VEGETABLE	Include at least one leafy green or yellow vegetable. Use the following fresh, cooked, canned, or frozen without salt: asparagus, broccoli, brussels sprouts, cabbage, cauliflower, chicory, cucumber, eggplant, endive, escarole, green beans, lettuce, mushrooms, okra, onions, pepper, pumpkin, radishes, rutabagas, squash, tomatoes, turnip greens, wax beans. Use fresh or canned peas only. Any vegetable which causes discomfort should be eliminated	Canned vegetables or juices, except low-sodium dietetic; any frozen vegetable processed with salt or sodium. Do not use these vegetables in any form: artichokes, beets, beet greens, carrots, celery, dandelion greens, kale, mustard greens, frozen peas and frozen lima beans, sauerkraut, spinach, white turnips
MISCELLANEOUS	Allspice, almond extract, basil, bay leaf, caraway, chives, cinnamon, cloves, coconut, curry, garlic, ginger, lemon juice, marjoram, mint, dry mustard, nutmeg, oregano, paprika, parsley, green pepper, peppermint extract, poultry seasoning, sage, sesame seeds, thyme, turmeric, vanilla extract, vinegar, unsalted peanut butter	Salted peanut butter, olives, pickles, relishes, ketchup, prepared mustard, garlic and celery salts, steak sauces, Worcestershire sauce, soy sauce, sodium additives, especially monosodium glutamate, patent medicines containing sodium, salt substitutes unless recommended by physician

SUGGESTED MEAL PATTERN

All foods must be prepared without salt or other sodium compounds such as monosodium glutamate.

BREAKFAST	Fruit or juice	1/2 cup
	Unsalted enriched cereal	1/2 cup
	Egg	1
	Unsalted bread	1 slice
	Unsalted butter or fortified margarine	1 tsp.
	Jelly	1 Tbsp.
	Sugar	1 tsp.

	Milk	1 cup
	Beverage	

LUNCH	Soup	1 cup
	Meat or substitute	2 ounces
	Potato or substitute	1/2 cup
	Vegetable	1/2 cup
	Salad, fruit	1/2 cup
	Unsalted salad dressing	1 Tbsp.
	Unsalted bread	1 slice
	Unsalted butter or fortified margarine	1 tsp.
	Fruit	1/2 cup
	Milk	1/2 cup
	Sugar	1 tsp.
	Beverage	

DINNER	Juice	1/2 cup
	Meat or substitute	2 ounces
	Potato or substitute	1/2 cup
	Vegetable	1/2 cup
	Salad, vegetable	3/4 cup
	Unsalted salad dressing	1 Tbsp.
	Unsalted bread	1 slice
	Unsalted butter or fortified margarine	1 tsp.
	Dessert	1/2 cup
	Milk	1/2 cup
	Sugar	1 tsp.
	Beverage	

FOR 250-MILLIGRAM SODIUM DIET (Approximately 11 mg. sodium) (Very severe restriction): Use 500-milligram Sodium Diet and substitute low-sodium milk for whole milk.

FOR 1,000-MILLIGRAM SODIUM DIET (Approximately 44 mg. sodium) (Moderate restriction). Use 500-Milligram Sodium Diet with any addition from the chart (on page 260) which will total an additional 500 milligrams.

*Based on material published by the American Heart Association on sodium-restricted diets.

** *Recipe for Low-Sodium Baking Powder:*

Potassium Bicarbonate	39.8 gm.
Cornstarch	28.0 gm.
Tartaric acid	7.5 gm.
Potassium Bitartrate	65.1 gm.

Substitute 1 1/2 teaspoons of this low-sodium baking powder for 1 teaspoon of regular baking powder.

2,000-Milligram Sodium Diet*
(Approximately 87 mg. of Sodium)

All foods must be prepared and served without salt.
Approximate Composition:

Calories: 1,900	Protein: 85 gm.
Fat: 63 gm.	Carbohydrate: 260 gm.
	Sodium: 2037 mg.

FOOD	TO INCLUDE	TO AVOID
BEVERAGE	Coffee, tea, cocoa, cereal beverage, carbonated beverages as allowed by physician. (For sodium content of specific beverages, see appendix)	Prepared beverage mixes, instant cocoa mixes, Dutch process cocoa, malted milk, fountain beverages
BREAD	Regular bread,* crackers with unsalted top. Limit bread to 3 slices daily	Bread or crackers made with baking powder, baking soda or salt; bread, crackers and rolls with salted tops
CEREAL	Enriched unsalted cooked cereal; dry cereals—1 serving daily	
CHEESE	¼ cup regular cottage cheese or 1 ounce of other natural unprocessed cheese (to be used in place of 1 ounce of meat or other substitutions as listed on chart)— otherwise, use low-salt or salt-free cheese	All other processed cheese
**DESSERT	Up to 1 prepared dessert per day to include regular plain cake, pudding, gelatin, etc. Milk used in desserts to be counted from day's allowance	Commercial sodium-containing gelatin desserts; desserts prepared with salt, baking powder, baking soda or egg white; pudding or cake mixes
EGG	One daily, if desired	None

---

* This is based on standard packaged bread—approximately 150 mg./slice. For bakery breads, rolls, and other specialty items—check manufacturer's calculation.
** This is based on a maximum of 300 mg. sodium per portion (as appears on labels). Note that bran cereals are higher in sodium than others.

FOOD	TO INCLUDE	TO AVOID
FAT	Up to 4 tsp. of salted butter or fortified margarine, commercial or home-prepared salad dressing, mayonnaise, sweet butter, salt-free margarine, and oil as desired	Salted butter or margarine in excess of allowed fat, commercial salad dressing prepared with salt or sodium
FRUIT	All fresh, canned, or frozen fruit and fruit juices, one of which is a source of vitamin C	Dried or canned fruit containing a sodium preservative
MEAT, FISH, FOWL	Limit to 6 ounces daily, all prepared without salt. Fresh fish or fish canned without salt, only; oysters, liver	Brains or kidneys; canned, salted, or smoked meat or fish, frozen fish, shellfish, except oysters
MILK	3 cups daily, including that used in cooking	All other
POTATO OR SUBSTITUTE	White or sweet potatoes, rice, corn, noodles, macaroni, dried peas, and lima beans	Potato chips
SOUP	Soup made from allowed foods	Canned, frozen, and dehydrated soup made with salt and bouillon in all forms
SWEETS	Sugar, honey, jellies, jams without sodium preservatives, homemade candy from allowed foods	Commercial candies and syrups, molasses, black licorice
VEGETABLE	Include at least one leafy green or yellow vegetable. All fresh, frozen, and unsalted canned vegetables	Canned vegetables or juices, except low-sodium dietetic; frozen peas and lima beans processed with salt or sodium; sauerkraut; salted canned tomato juice; tomatoes; and tomato sauce
MISCELLANEOUS	Allspice, almond extract, basil, bay leaf, caraway, chives, cinnamon, cloves, coconut, curry, garlic, ginger, lemon juice, marjoram, mint, dry	Salted peanut butter, olives, pickles, relishes, ketchup, prepared mustard, garlic and celery salts, steak sauces, Worcestershire sauce, soy

FOOD	*TO INCLUDE*	*TO AVOID*
	mustard, nutmeg, oregano, paprika, parsley, green pepper, peppermint extract, poultry seasoning, sage, sesame seeds, thyme, turmeric, vanilla extract, vinegar, unsalted peanut butter	sauce, sodium additives, especially monosodium glutamate; patent medicines containing sodium, salt substitutes unless recommended by physician

Suggested Meal Pattern

All foods must be prepared and served without salt or other sodium compounds such as monosodium glutamate.

BREAKFAST	Fruit or juice	1/2 cup
	Enriched cereal	1/2 cup
	Egg	1
	Salted bread	1 slice
	Unsalted butter or fortified margarine	1 tsp.
	Jelly	1 Tbsp.
	Sugar	3 tsp.
	Milk—whole	1 cup
	Beverage	
LUNCH	Soup (made from foods allowed)	1 cup
	Meat or substitute*	2 ounces
	Potato or substitute	1/2 cup
	Vegetable	1/2 cup
	Salted salad dressing	1 Tbsp.
	Salted bread	1 slice
	Unsalted butter or fortified margarine	1 tsp.
	Fruit	1/2 cup
	Milk—whole	1 cup
	Sugar	2 tsp.
	Beverage	
DINNER	Juice	1/2 cup
	Meat or substitute	3 ounces
	Potato or substitute	1/2 cup
	Vegetable	1/2 cup
	Salad, vegetable	3/4 cup
	Oil and vinegar dressing	1 Tbsp.
	Salted bread	1 slice
	Unsalted butter or fortified margarine	1 tsp.
	Dessert	1/2 cup
	Milk—whole	1 cup
	Sugar	2 tsp.
	Beverage	

* 1/2 cup of cottage cheese: 2% fat was used.

No-Added-Salt Diet
(Approximately 4,000 Milligrams Sodium)

This diet provides a mild restriction in sodium by using the regular diet and omitting highly salted foods and the use of salt at the table. One-half (1/2) teaspoon of salt is allowed daily for food preparation (One-half [1/2] teaspoon of salt = approximately 1,000 mg. sodium).

Approximate Composition:

Calories: 1800	Protein: 77 gm.
Fat: 62 gm.	Carbohydrate: 238 gm.

FOOD	TO INCLUDE	TO AVOID
BEVERAGE	All	None
CEREAL	All enriched or whole grain, except those to avoid	Bread, crackers, and rolls with salted toppings, pretzels
CHEESE	1 ounce mild American or Swiss, 1/4 cup lightly salted cottage, pot, or ricotta	Aged and processed cheese and cheese spreads
DESSERT	All varieties, but not more than 1 pastry-type per day	None
EGG	One daily	Note limitation in amount
FAT	Butter and fortified margarine, cream, oil, french dressing, mayonnaise	Bacon and bacon fat, salt pork
FRUIT	All—one of which is a source of vitamin C	None
MEAT, FISH, FOWL	All fresh, frozen, or canned	Highly salted or smoked: corned beef, ham, hash, spam, frankfurters, lox, and kippers
MILK	3 cups daily	Note limitation in amount
POTATO OR SUBSTITUTE	All except potato chips	Potato chips
SOUP	All homemade soup, with permitted ingredients; low-sodium bouillon	Bouillon in all forms, meat extracts, canned, frozen, and dehydrated soup
SWEETS	All except black licorice	Black licorice
VEGETABLE	All fresh, frozen, or canned, except those to avoid. Include one leafy green or yellow vegetable at least 4 times weekly	Sauerkraut or other vegetables prepared in brine

FOOD	TO INCLUDE	TO AVOID
MISCELLANEOUS	All except those to avoid	Peanut butter; olives; ketchup; celery, onion, and garlic salts, except in place of regular salt; chili sauce; horseradish; meat sauces; meat extracts; monosodium glutamate; prepared mustard; pickles; relishes; soy sauce; Worcestershire sauce; steak sauce; patent medicine containing sodium

* Based on material published by The American Heart Association on sodium-restricted diets.

Suggested Meal Pattern

Do not use salt at the table. One-half (1/2) teaspoon salt allowed daily for food preparation.

BREAKFAST	Fruit or juice	1/2 cup
	Cereal	1/2 cup
	Egg	1
	Bread	1 slice
	Butter or fortified margarine	1 tsp.
	Jelly	1 Tbsp.
	Sugar	1 tsp.
	Milk	1 cup
	Beverage	
LUNCH	Soup	1 cup
	Meat or substitute	2 ounces
	Potato or substitute	1/2 cup
	Vegetable	1/2 cup
	Salad, vegetable	3/4 cup
	Salad dressing	1 Tbsp.
	Bread	1 slice
	Butter or fortified margarine	1 tsp.
	Fruit	1/2 cup
	Milk	1/2 cup
	Sugar	1 tsp.
	Beverage	
DINNER	Fruit or juice	1/2 cup
	Meat or substitute	3 ounces
	Potato or substitute	1/2 cup
	Vegetable	1/2 cup
	Salad, fruit	1/2 cup

Salad dressing	1 Tbsp.
Bread	1 slice
Butter or fortified margarine	1 tsp.
Dessert	1/2 cup
Milk	1/2 cup
Sugar	1 tsp.
Beverage	

▪ *Notes* ▪

Chapter 1   WHAT IN THE WORLD CAN I EAT?
1. Jean Carper, *The Food Pharmacy* (New York: Bantam Books, 1988), 57.

Chapter 2   THE ANTI-CANCER DIET
1. Nina Killham (of the *Washington Post*), "Nutritional Changes Advocated in the Fight Against Breast Cancer; National Women's Health Network Seeks to Promote a Low-Fat Diet as a Strategy to Lowering Risks and Curbing Spread of the Deadly Disease," *Los Angeles Times*, 3 Sept. 1987.
2. Carol Krucoff, "Cancer in the Mind of America; Poll Finds Widespread Dread, and Some Steps Toward Prevention," *Washington Post*, 30 Sept. 1986.
3. Dr. Richard Rivlin, Dr. Peter Greenwald, and Dr. Charles LeMaistre, as quoted by Karen Wilk Rubin, "Diet and Cancer," *Restaurant Business*, 1 March 1988.
4. Jane E. Brody (of the National Cancer Institute), "Personal Health: Sorting Out Data on Diet and Cancer," *New York Times*, 30 Sept. 1987.
5. Cheryl Loggins, "No Single Food Can Prevent Disease; Total Diet Is Key to Protecting Good Health," *Los Angeles Times*, 26 June 1986.
6. Killham, op. cit.
7. Ibid.
8. Ibid.
9. Sally Squires, "An Ounce of Prevention; How to Reduce Your Risk of Getting Cancer," *Washington Post*, 30 Sept. 1986.
10. John Dickerson, "Less Fat in Diet Could Help Prevent Breast Cancer," Xinhua News Agency, 29 April 1987.
11. Squires, op. cit.
12. Gayle Young, "UPI Science: Your Health—The Mystique of Fiber," United Press International, 8 Feb. 1987.
13. Ibid.
14. Ibid.
15. "Nutrients Found Lung Cancer Curb," *New York Times*, 13 Nov. 1986, Sec. 2, 11:1.
16. Rob Stein, "Vitamins May Help Prevent Lung Cancer," United Press International, 13 Nov. 1986.
17. Dr. Emily White, "Medical Experts Report Progress Against Colorectal Cancer," *Business Wire*, 31 Oct. 1986.
18. Dr. Tim Byers, "Cancer," United Press International, 25 June 1987.
19. Cheryl Loggins, "Link Between Diet and Disease Prevention Called Exaggerated; Evidence Is Lacking to Prove that Certain Foods Can Prevent Specific Health Ailments," *Los Angeles Times*, 22 Jan. 1987.
20. Kathleen McAuliffe, "New Research Theory: To Prevent Cancer, Count Your Calories," *U.S. News & World Report*, 10 March 1986, 67–68.
21. Carole Sugarman, Tom Sietsema, "Food: Flashes in the Pan," *Washington Post*, 1 April 1987.
22. Ibid.
23. Ibid.

Chapter 3 ANTI-HEART ATTACK DIET
1. Joanne Silberner, "New Blast at Cholesterol; Simpler Ground Rules May Make It Easier to Cut the Fat—and Live Longer," *U.S. News & World Report,* 19 Oct. 1987, 76–77.
2. Ibid.
3. Ibid.
4. Lee Siegel, "Food Chemicals, New Type of Egg Can Control Heart-Threatening Cholesterol," Associated Press, 3 May 1988.
5. Silberner, op. cit.
6. Patricia Picone Mitchell, "The Sad Truth About Dieting; The More Often You Lose, the Less Likely You'll Win," *Washington Post,* 27 May 1987, E16.
7. "Diet-Exercise Program Rates as Best Way to Lose Weight," *Los Angeles Times,* 23 March, 1986.
8. Amy Mednick, "Rating Pros, Cons of Fish Oil Supplements," *Los Angeles Times,* 28 Oct. 1986, 4.
9. Ibid.
10. Mary A. Dempsey, "Young Women Are Neglected Heart Attack Group," United Press International, 10 Oct. 1986.

Chapter 4 ANTI-STROKE DIET
1. Charles S. Taylor, "Doctors Tout Benefits of High Fiber, Low Fat Diet," United Press International, 17 Oct. 1986.
2. "Diet-Exercise Program Rates as Best Way to Lose Weight," *Los Angeles Times,* 13 March 1986.
3. Ralph E. Minear, M.D., *The Joy of Living Salt-Free,* (New York: Macmillan, 1984).
4. *Health Letter,* Harvard University School of Medicine, 1979.

Chapter 5 EXERCISE AND YOUR HEALTH
1. Patricia Picone Mitchell, "The Sad Truth About Dieting; The More Often You Lose, the Less Likely You'll Win," *Washington Post,* 27 May 1987, E16.
2. "Running: Good for the Soul, Too?" *The New York Times,* 15 Feb. 1988, II, 11:1.
3. Ibid.

▪ *Index* ▪